Pocket Picture Guides

Recognition of Child Abuse and Neglect

Stephen J. Rose
MA, MB, B Chir, MRCP

Lecturer in Paediatrics
University of Aberdeen
Aberdeen, UK

Gower Medical Publishing · London · New York · 1985

© Copyright 1985 by Gower Medical Publishing Ltd.
34-42 Cleveland Street, London W1P 5FB, England.
All rights reserved. No part of this publication may be
reproduced, stored in a retrieval system or transmitted in
any form or by any means electronic, mechanical,
photocopying, recording or otherwise, without prior
written permission of the publisher.

Distribution limited to United Kingdom.

ISBN 0-906923-41-7

British Library Cataloguing in Publication Data
Rose, Stephen J.
    Recognition of child abuse and neglect. –
    (Pocket picture guides to clinical medicine; v.7)
    1. Battered child syndrome
    I. Title   II. Series
    617'.1'0088054   RA1122.5

Project Editor: Fiona Carr
    Designer: Teresa Foster

Printed in Italy by Imago Publishing Ltd.

Contents

To my Wife
Beatriz

Acknowledgements
I would like to acknowledge the encouragement, support
and critical assessment freely given by Professor D.
Barltrop, Professor of Child Health, Westminster Medical
School, London and Dr. C. A. S. Galloway, Consultant
Paediatrician, Raigmore Hospital, Inverness. I would
also like to thank them and Professor A. G. M. Campbell,
Professor of Child Health, University of Aberdeen for the
use of much of the illustrative material. Professor S. R.
Meadow, Professor of Child Health, University of Leeds,
kindly provided the case histories of the deliberate
poisoning of children by their parents. Finally, I would
like to thank the publishers for their continual faith in the
project.

Introduction

Non-accidental injury (NAI) has been the subject of a multiplicity of papers and texts over the last two decades. Much is now known of the psychological and social factors which predispose to 'baby-battering' and the caring professions are alert to the recognition of injury. There can be few, therefore, who fail to recognise gross forms of physical and psychological abuse. However, so much pressure has recently been exerted on medical and social workers to identify all children 'at risk' that it is not uncommon to encounter parents who have suffered the humiliating experience of being unjustly accused of abusing their children. Others have been subjected to an unexplained increase in surveillance because of suspicion of battering.

The purpose of this book is to elucidate some of the difficulties in differentiating early signs of NAI from medical problems which may resemble or mimic abuse.

The early detection of NAI may save further suffering and possibly prevent death, but much depends upon the informed observer, as children less than three years old are unable to express their fears, and older children may be reluctant to do so. NAI may be either physical or psychological, and the latter (the so-called 'soft-battering') may be extremely difficult to detect as abnormal behaviour may emerge only after abuse has continued for a considerable time.

It is important to recognise the episodic character of the problem. There is usually a premonitory phase during which the parent struggles for self-control. At this time the child may exhibit signs of malnutrition, failure to thrive and general physical neglect. It is easy to describe the 'typical' battering parent: a young, unmarried and isolated mother with no family support, on inadequate income, attempting to contend with a difficult and demanding infant. It must be remembered, however, that most parents in this 'stereotyped' situation will not injure their children, and, conversely, that battering also occurs in respectable, high-income, stable environments. Also NAI may be caused by persons other than the parents, e.g. baby-sitters, cohabitees, siblings and even pets!

1

Multiple injuries of different ages are alerting, and suspicion will be enhanced if an inadequate explanation is offered, or if there appears to be parental indifference. In cases of NAI, explanations may be inconsistent with the age of the child or with the site and nature of the injury. There may well be discrepancies with previous explanations which may be excessively vague, extremely detailed or sometimes entirely improbable.

It should be remembered, however, that a generally inarticulate person may offer a vague explanation even if it is true. A minor injury should be noted if there has been a series of poorly explained injuries to the child, or if there is any suspicion of battering of the siblings.

Many social and psychological factors have been indentified as increasing the risk of battering and the more factors applicable to the situation, the higher the likelihood of battering. The stability of the marriage is an important factor, as is a drink or drug problem, record of violence on the part of either parent or if the parents themselves were battered. A psychiatric history or a personality disorder relating to either parent also lends weight to any suspicion.

It is interesting to note that battering is more common among infants who have been separated from their mother at birth, but if a child is breast-fed for more than five weeks, battering is rare.

Psychological battering is far more difficult to detect and will probably only become apparent when the victim is unable to cope anymore, and this may be weeks or months after the inception of the abuse.

The younger child may fail to thrive, become withdrawn, unstable or depressed and refuse to be comforted or cuddled by adults. If he becomes fearful of his parents he may well treat all adults with suspicion. He will withdraw, but watch alertly, without expression as if expecting the next blow. Such an expression is called 'frozen awareness' (Fig. 1). The neglected child may be excessively friendly towards strangers and demand attention from everybody. The school-age child may also withdraw, and become depressed, allow academic standards to fall and become indifferent towards achievement, especially if the family place emphasis on success, but ignore emotional requirements. In extreme cases, the older child or adolescent may attempt suicide.

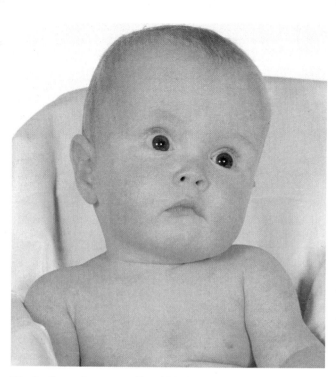

Fig. 1 Frozen Awareness. The child who only sees his parents to be assaulted, comes to view all adults with suspicion. There is no spontaneous smile or reaction when he sees an adult, indeed, he may withdraw into a corner and start screaming in anticipation of the pain. Eventually, this reaction is controlled and the child remains expressionless, but alert and watchful. This child shows such an expression. His eyes are alert and he has fixed on an object, but his face remains totally dead-pan, registering neither interest, nor happiness, nor fear.

Incest

The incidence of incest is unknown, but it is probably not uncommon. It has been suggested that 75% of paedophilia cases are incestuous. Incest rarely involves physical violence and therefore detectable physical signs are rare, especially as much incest involves genital viewing, fondling or oro-genital stimulation involving no genital injury. The vast majority of victims are female, the commonest liaison being between step-father and step-daughter. The abuse often commences when the victim is aged eight to ten years, although no age-group is immune.

The psychological effects may be similar to those seen in 'soft-battering'. If the child is less than five years old, there may be signs of developmental repression or regression with inappropriate and excessive clinging to the parents, and frequent night-terrors. In the older child, these may be school failure, weight loss or gain, depression or conversion hysteria. Finally the child may run away from home. Obviously, by the time any of these signs are detectable, gross psychological disturbance has occurred.

Whenever any form of non-accidental injury is suspected, many factors must be taken into consideration before any accusation or hint of accusation is levelled.

Bruises and Assaults

Bruises are virtually universal in the mobile child. A recent survey of nursery school children revealed that all had bruises, many of which were of different ages, an often quoted feature of non-accidental injury (NAI). Much normal bruising occurs over bony prominences or on unprotected areas, such as the head, back and limbs (Fig. 2). However, because these areas are unprotected, they may be implicated in NAI (Figs. 3–6). Medical causes frequently mimic bruising (Figs. 7 and 8) or it can be caused by a bleeding tendency (Figs. 9, 10 and 12). Bruising on the immobile child is cause for concern, as is bruising in unusual places which are either protected or not over bony prominences. The neck (Figs. 14 and 15) is normally protected, and the ample musculature of the buttocks cushions blows, so that bruising requires force (Fig. 17). The genital area in both sexes is well protected so any lesions in this area (Figs. 20–26) require explanation. Symmetrically arranged bruising on the back (Fig. 27) may indicate that the child has been picked up and squeezed or shaken. Many parents are unaware that shaking an infant can cause serious damage, such as fractured ribs or a subdural haemorrhage (Fig. 79), which may result in mental retardation or possibly death.

Black eyes in the immobile child (Fig. 30) are rarely accidental, although one must be wary of medical causes (Figs. 31–34). In the mobile child, black eyes are a common sequel to childhood aggression, but equally may result from an adult assault (Fig. 35). Two black eyes are associated with fracture of the base of the skull, which requires considerable force, such as in a road traffic accident, but they are more likely to be the result of an assault (Fig. 36). A black eye results from direct trauma to the surrounding tissues, whereas a blow on the head, distant from the eye, can cause a subconjunctival haemorrhage (Figs. 37, 78).

Multiple injuries offer grounds for suspicion (Figs. 5, 27, 38) especially if the lesions are of different ages. However, the importance of gaining an overall view is demonstrated by the case of a father accused of assaulting his son who had finger marks on one arm and bruising on the side of his face. The father explained that he had grabbed the child's arm on seeing him about to fall from a chair, thus causing the child to swing round and hit his face on the seat of the chair. This explanation was disbelieved but the father was eventually exonerated, only after extensive questioning of himself, his wife and his neighbours, causing considerable discomfiture to the family and embarrassment to the investigator.

The shape of an injury may be helpful; if clearly distinguishable, such as finger marks (Figs. 17, 27, 38) or belt or whip marks (Fig. 39), the observer should be alert to the possibility of an assault. Injuries with straight edges (Figs. 41, 42, 44, 46) are unlikely to have been caused accidentally. As a general rule, straight lines are 'man made' whereas irregular lines are 'natural'. Sadly, even the maxim is challenged medically (Figs. 43 and 45).

Bites (Figs. 5 and 47) are commonly inflicted on children by their peers or pets (Fig. 48) and are frequently distinctive. However, it is important to take careful note of the size and shape of the bite marks, to determine the likelihood of this being sibling rivalry or something more sinister.

Bruising around the mouth (Figs. 50 and 85) may be significant, especially if the frenulum of the upper lip or tongue is torn. This can occur during a 'feeding battle' or when something is rammed into the child's mouth to stop it crying. Derangement of the teeth (Fig. 51) requires considerable force and demands a plausible explanation.

Bruising is the hallmark of the active child and this, combined with the many similar looking medical conditions, make the distinction of the battered child from the normal, unnervingly difficult.

Careful consideration of all factors, physical and social, is mandatory. The explanation of the injuries must be compatible with those injuries: is there an appropriate degree of concern? Too much concern can have the same connotations as indifference. Has medical advice been sought if it is indicated, or has there been an attempt to cover up? Any previous history of battering, whether of that child or a sibling should be elicited, from outside sources if necessary. It can be seen from the foregoing text that attempting to isolate the non-accidental bruising is fraught with pitfalls. Aspects of the bruising which may help are the site, the shape, the number of bruises and whether they are of different ages.

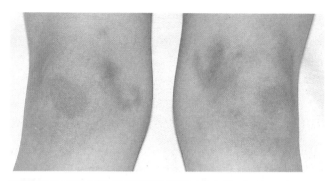

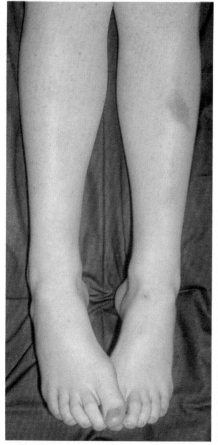

Fig. 2 Normal bruises. Mobile children are constantly acquiring bruises. These may result from collisions, peer battles, falls from bikes; the possibilities are endless. Normal bruising, therefore, tends to occur over bony, vulnerable surfaces such as the forehead, shins and back, or, in childhood battles, the face. A physically active or aggressive child may sport multiple bruises of different ages which can be features of non-accidental injury. The family method of correction may be spanking using the hand, slipper or belt. If this leaves bruising, is it excessive or acceptable? It is obvious, therefore, that to use bruising as the main criterion for deciding whether a child should stay with the family or not, is fraught with hazards.

7

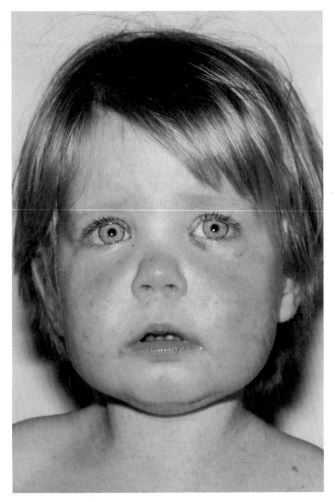

Fig. 3 Non-accidental bruising. The face is frequently bruised. The toddler judges the height of objects poorly and uses the forehead as a testing device. Objects at the level of the eyes are normally avoided, so bruising on the lower face is less common. Conversely the face is picked out as the target in childhood battles. Parental displeasure may be displayed as violence, and slaps across the face may be harder than intended if tempers fray, or the parents have been drinking. This child has extensive bruising on both cheeks with accompanying scratches. There is little doubt that this child has been assaulted; the detection of the perpetrator could be far more difficult.

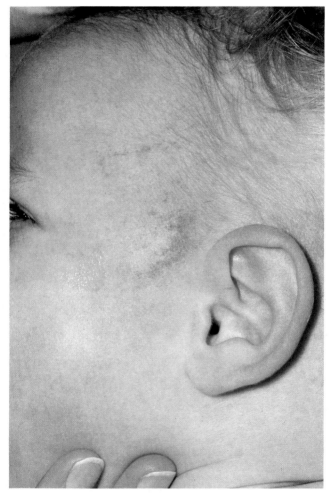

Fig. 4 Non-accidental bruising. The non-walking child is not prone to self-inflicted injury except scratching. The child is not strong enough to cause bruising and falls from the sitting position are less likely to cause damage than those from the standing position. This site of bruising, in front of the ear, is common, as the skin is easily crushed against the underlying bone. The bruising is extensive, extending up onto the temple and, as the child is young, he is unlikely to have sufficient power to inflict such damage himself. Further examination of this child revealed the bruising seen in Fig. 14. This combination heightens the suspicion of NAI.

9

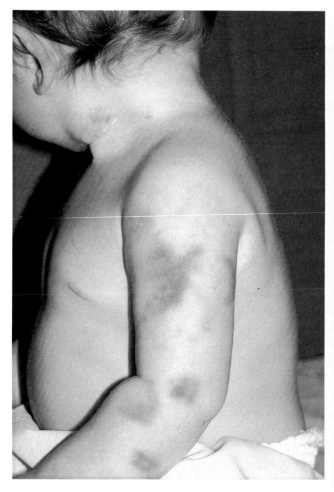

Fig. 5 Non-accidental injury. This child bears evidence of multiple injuries: there is bruising on the arm, around the neck and a suspicion of a bite mark on the upper arm. All the injuries appear to be of the same age, suggesting a frenzied attack, inflicting multiple injuries. It is difficult to give an accidental explanation for such an appearance in a non-walking child and assault is a more plausible explanation. This is also suggested by the bite mark, which cannot be accidental, although it could be produced by an enraged or jealous sibling. It is important to study the shape, distribution and age of all marks and this may help differentiate the accidentally and non-accidentally injured child.

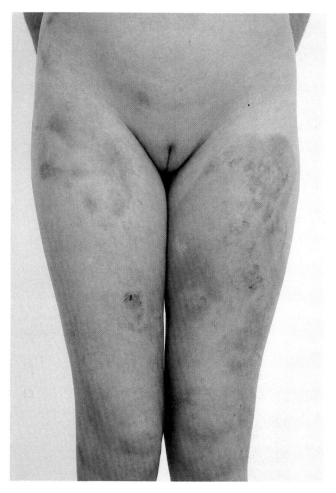

Fig. 6 Non-accidental bruising. The buttocks and thighs are well muscled and may be amply covered with fat. These areas tend to be cushioned from blows, so bruising requires more force than over other areas of skin. This child has extensive bruising over the thighs and extending onto the abdomen. No individual marks can be identified which suggests a severe beating with the resultant injuries merging with each other. Such bruising, interspersed with multiple abrasions is not likely to have been caused by accident or peer group battles. A deliberate excessive assault is the most likely explanation.

11

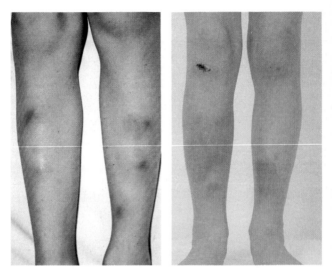

Fig. 7   Skin lesions (Erythema nodosum). This skin disease accompanies many childhood illnesses, especially those which are infective, either as part of the disease process or as a result of treatment. It may occur with bacterial, viral or fungal diseases, certain bowel problems or as a side-effect of many drugs including some commonly prescribed antibiotics. It may also evolve spontaneously; adolescent boys being the commonest affected group. The lesions mimic bruises closely, they usually start as red areas on the skin, then darken centrally (left) and eventually look like bruising (right). The affected areas are tender, usually more so than bruising, and there may be no explanation for their sudden occurrence.

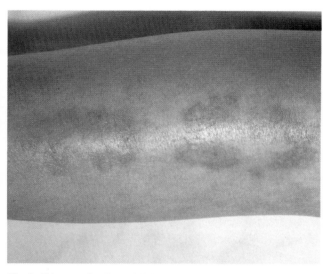

Fig. 8 Skin complications of diabetes mellitus. This skin problem is a rare accompaniment to diabetes mellitus and is seen more frequently in adults than children. As this is a rare condition, it is not well known, either by parents of diabetic children or the lay public, so that the sudden appearance of such skin changes, mimicking bruising, will not be easily explained. Fortunately, both this lesion and the previous (Fig. 7) occur on the shins, so are less likely to attract much attention. However, in the child who is already under surveillance, they may be marked down as yet another unexplained injury.

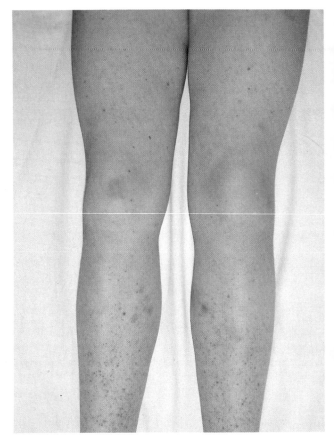

Fig. 9 Bleeding disorder. Bleeding disorders may be inherited, such as haemophilia, or be caused by an acquired lack of clotting factors, either from destruction or from excessive usage. The child is then at risk from excessive bleeding after minor injury or spontaneous bleeding. This may occur into the skin, as here, causing bruising, into the internal organs, causing pain suggesting internal damage, or, most seriously, into the head, causing nerve damage and loss of consciousness. Thus damage usually caused by NAI may occur spontaneously in a child with a bleeding tendency. Such children are exceptional and the explanation that the child bruises easily is rarely true. This child is suffering from a lack of platelets which plug the otherwise leaky minute blood vessels. This is a common disorder which can occur after infective childhood illnesses. It causes the very small bleeding points seen on the lower leg, which do not occur in NAI and can be used as a differentiating point.

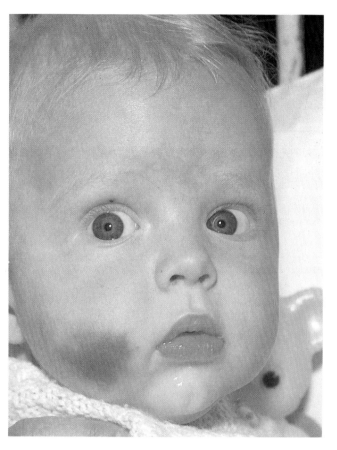

Fig. 10 Haemophilia. This young child has an extensive bruise on the lower jaw, an injury more consistent with deliberate assault than accident, especially as the child is not yet walking. However, minor trauma, such as turning the head suddenly and colliding with a hard object, can cause extensive bleeding in a child with haemophilia. There are different degrees of severity of the disease; the most severe causes spontaneous bleeding and is often noted shortly after birth. Children with the less severe forms may bruise easily with extensive bleeding but have few additional symptoms. These children may not be taken to the doctor for diagnosis, so can be seen with extensive bruising and an explanation which could not suffice for such bruising in a normal child.

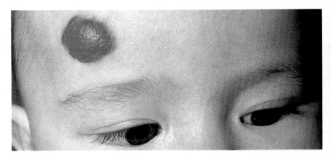

Fig. 11 Birthmark (strawberry naevus). Birthmarks are common and vary in their appearance (Figs. 21, 22 (lower), 33, 49). The strawberry naevus, so named because of its colour and texture, is very common. The infant is born either with no skin problems or a small defect and the naevus grows during the first months of life. Reference to old photographs may not reveal any such problem. The naevi are often multiple and of different sizes. They are not tender, feel soft and fleshy and remain constant for weeks, unlike a bruise. The results of an assault are invariably painful, allowing differentiation.

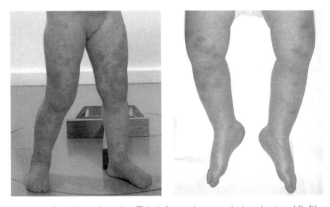

Fig. 12 Bleeding disorder. This infant, who can obviously stand (left) but has a tottering gait, has lower limbs covered in bruises. Even with unstable bipedal progression, such bruising is unlikely to have occurred accidentally. Similarly it is difficult to explain such a pattern, with large numbers of discrete bruises, occurring from deliberate attack. If the parents are unable to furnish an acceptable explanation, the observer must be able to make an informed guess at the fashion of deliberate assault. It is unjustifiable to assume that an implausible or absent explanation necessarily implies NAI. This child also has an acute transient bleeding disorder, producing spontaneous bruising in the poorly mobile child. This is seen more vividly in the child on the right where the infant is not walking, but sports multiple bruises.

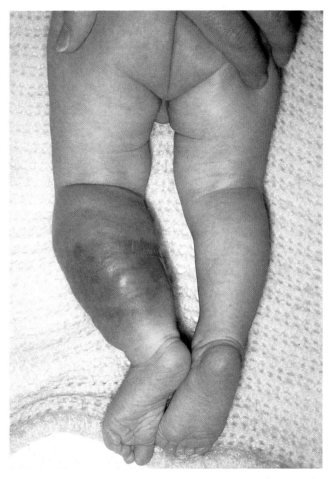

Fig. 13 Blood vessel malformation. This fiery, painful-looking area of the lower leg is a developmental abnormality of blood vessels. Unlike the strawberry naevus, this defect would have been present at birth, although changes may occur with growth. Old photographs are thus more helpful if doubts arise. If this lesion was due to bruising or possibly infection, the child would be miserable, the area, exquisitely tender and the infant would probably refuse to move the limb. Gentle examination of a child is possible without causing undue pain, even if injured, and this may enable differentiation between painless congenital abnormalities and painful trauma.

17

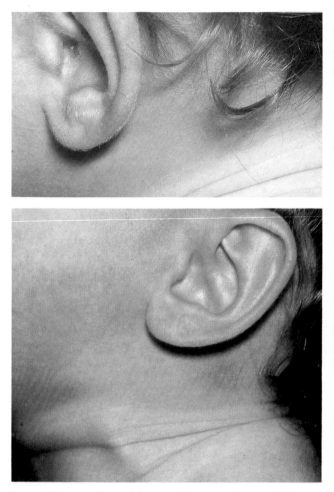

Fig.14 Bruising of the neck. The neck is a protected area of the body; the force of most collisions being taken either on the head or chest. Even the toddler generally manages to avoid contact with objects at eye level or lower but the forehead does not fare so well. Accidental damage could possibly occur if the child fell sideways onto an object, but even this is unlikely to cause such extensive bruising. Although this child has marked bruising, there are no finger marks, suggesting that this damage did not result from gripping the child. A vicious blow is more likely, either from a considerably older sibling or an adult. Even if this were the only injury in the child, it is alerting and a plausible explanation must be sought.

18

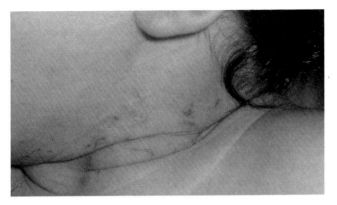

Fig. 15 Scratch marks around the neck. Self-inflicted scratch marks appear at an early age. The random movements of the newborn infant frequently cause scratch marks, especially of the face. As the child's movements become more co-ordinated, then scratching becomes reserved for dealing with itches, which tend to be localised. Extensive scratches, as in this figure, are not likely to be self-inflicted. Conceivably, a pet, such as a cat could inflict such damage, but an outside human agent appears to be the most likely perpetrator. Scratch marks around an infant's neck is rather a curious injury and if NAI is contemplated, an explanation for this damage must be offered by the observer.

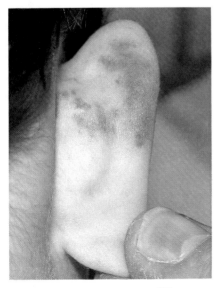

Fig. 16 Bruising of the ear. Bruising in this area is common in the older child. The ear is soft and easily crushed against the hard surface of the skull. 'Cauliflower' ears are the result of pugilism, or contact sports. A blow on the ear may also be the accepted form of correction. An isolated bruise in such an exposed area as this is of no value in detecting the battered child. However, repeated similar bruising may be sufficient to alert the careful observer.

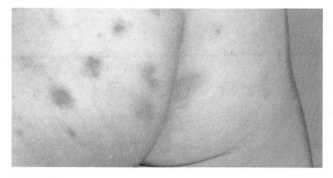

Fig. 17 Finger marks on buttocks. The muscle and fat of the buttocks cushion blows so that bruising requires considerable force. Even corrective spanking only leaves a reddened sore bottom which rapidly returns to normal. This child has multiple small bruises on the buttocks, which are very like finger marks, the thumb marks being near the natal cleft. The bruising itself is neither severe nor extensive and would not warrant suspicion. However, the recognisable finger prints imply deliberate injury. It is important to examine the shape of the bruising, which may be more worrying than the extent.

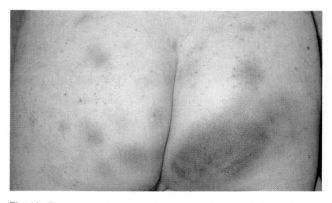

Fig. 18 Bleeding disorder. The damage to this child's buttocks is more horrifying than that in Fig. 17. There are multiple bruises, of different ages and an extensive bruise on one buttock. There are, however, no recognisable shapes or patterns to the bruising. This child suffers from a more severe form of haemophilia, which allows marked bleeding, and thus bruising, to occur after minor trauma only. The large bruise overlies the area of greatest pressure when the child is sitting, so an unexpected topple backwards with a subsequent hard landing would be sufficient to cause this extensive bruise. This child is likely to have bruising elswhere, from repeated trauma which may help the diagnosis or may be misinterpreted as repeated assault.

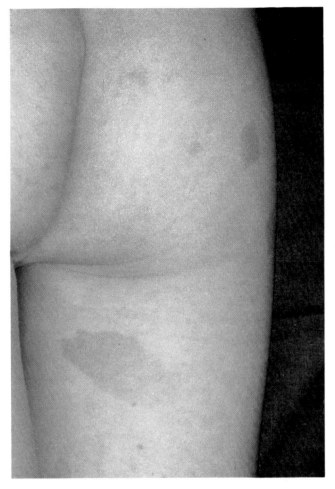

Fig. 19 Skin pigmentation. Increased skin pigmentation, such as moles, is associated with increasing age, however, light brown marks called 'café au lait' spots are very common in childhood. One or two occur in many children and several diseases are associated with these spots, which may be the first indication of the underlying disease. The spots vary in size and shape, are irregular, and can resemble fading bruises. The colour of the spots is uniform in any child, suggesting all resulted from a single 'assault'. However, these skin lesions are not tender and do not change with time, as would be expected with bruising.

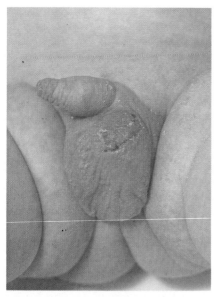

Fig. 20 Non-accidental injury. The genital area in both sexes is well protected and, as the organs are soft, bruising will only occur if crushed against the surrounding bone. If the child is not walking, any damage in this area, unless part of a nappy rash, is likely to have been inflicted by outside agents. The genital area is tender and need never be on public display, so deliberate injury would cause considerable pain, yet remain undetected.

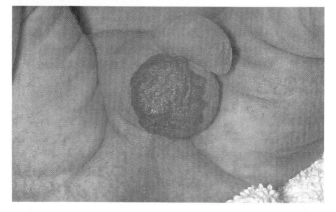

Fig. 21 Strawberry naevus. These blood vessel malformations can occur anywhere in the body and alter with time. Initially they enlarge, then become static, then resolve from the centre outwards (Fig. 49). Despite the brilliant red implied by their name, their colour can be darker and mimic bruising. The naevus shown here is painless and has a raised edge so that the distinction between normal and abnormal tissue is easily felt. Although the centre of a bruise is obvious, the edges are indistinct and the swollen tissues merge imperceptibly into the surrounding normal tissue.

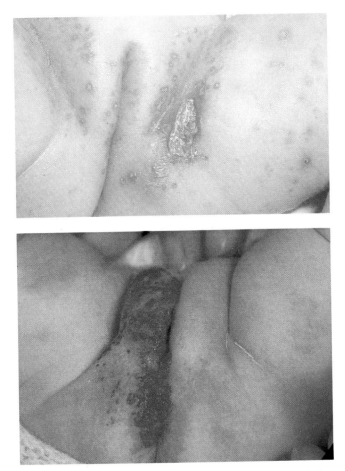

Fig. 22 Pubic skin lesions. The pubic area is commonly implicated in nappy rashes causing areas of inflammation, infection and, occasionally, frank ulceration (top). This child has a punched out ulcer in the skin fold, an area usually spared by nappy rash, and little evidence of a skin rash on the buttocks. This has the hallmark of NAI, but the child has had a serious illness and the ulcer resulted from loss of blood supply to that area secondary to blockage of the blood vessels. The child recovered and returned home and the ulcer healed slowly. Hospital admissions are normally rapidly relayed to the primary care physician to whom reference should be made if doubt exists. The child in the lower picture has a strawberry naevus of the vulva, which mimics a recent bruise. Methods for differentiating this from injury are previously described (Figs. 11 and 21).

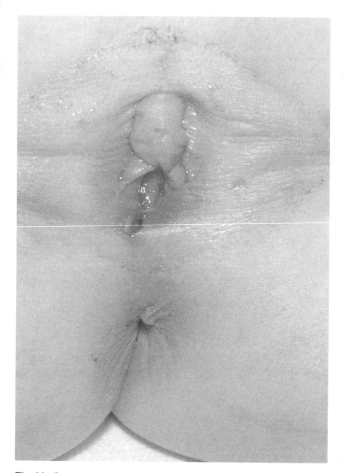

Fig. 23 Sexual assault. The commonest form of sexual assault on children is incest and the commonest liaison is between step-father and step-daughter, however, all combinations occur. Straddle injuries in a girl, such as falling across a bar, will cause bruising to the vulva as well as vagina, but here the vulva is spared, suggesting direct assault. This bruising will have been caused by an erect penis or finger; if the hymen (maidenhead) is torn, penetration has occurred. The child may have no other evidence of injury, but even minor damage in this area should be regarded with grave suspicion. The victim of incest will frequently not complain, indeed, she may consider it a normal part of family behaviour; such children are therefore highly difficult to detect, and may be discovered only after the incestuous relationship has continued for years.

24

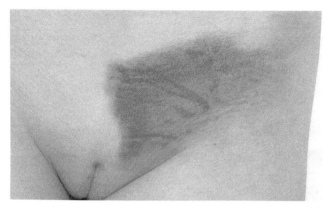

Fig. 24 Non-accidental injury. Although the bruising in this figure is also in the pubic area, it does not have the same sexual connotations as the bruising in Fig. 23. This bruising may have resulted from a kick, for example. Bruising in this area is uncommon accidentally, especially in girls, who partake in contact sports less commonly. The usual accidental genital bruising occurs from straddling injuries. This bruise also has definite straight line edges, not a feature of accidental bruising. Such an injury requires a plausible explanation and should otherwise be viewed with suspicion.

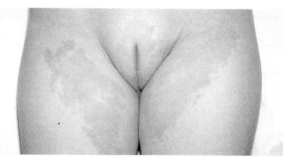

Fig. 25 Urticaria (hives). Allergic children frequently manifest their allergy as a skin lesion, especially when the allergy is to a foodstuff such as chocolate, strawberries or shellfish. This is known as urticaria, which, in the acute phase, can mimic the redness produced by slap marks. In this child, slapping across the thighs and genital area could have sexual connotations and so should not be suggested without substantial evidence. The urticaria is also extremely itchy inducing intense scratching. The redness disappears within a matter of hours possibly leaving the child with extensive scratching for no apparent reason and an explanation for which the evidence has just disappeared.

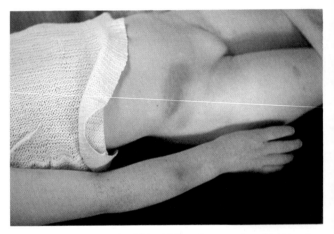

Fig. 26 Bleeding disorder. This child has the same transient bleeding disorder as the child shown in Fig. 9. There is a deficiency in the platelet plugs allowing leakage from the blood vessels. The bruising is near the pubic area, but significantly is over a bony prominence, the rim of the pelvic bone. This is a common site for bruising and minor trauma in this girl would cause the extensive bruising seen. Interestingly, she has very few of the small pin-point haemorrhages which are characteristic of a platelet deficiency.

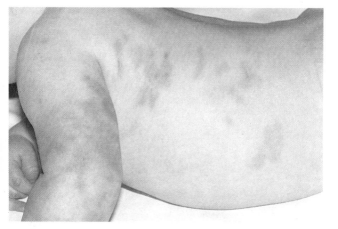

Fig. 27 Multiple grip marks. Shaking is a common method of attempting to quieten the child or relieve frustration. The child is picked up by the chest so that finger marks are seen parallel to the spine and longitudinal finger marks are seen on the side of the chest as in this figure. This child has probably been gripped twice around the chest and also by the arms. The child is shaken back and forth violently which may fracture ribs, cause a subconjunctival haemorrhage (Fig. 37) or produce bleeding into the skull (subdural haematoma Fig. 79). Obvious finger marks such as these do not occur during normal play, even if this includes tossing the child into the air and catching him around the chest. Such marks require considerable pressure.

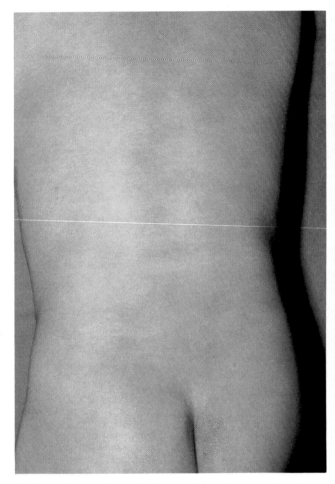

Fig. 28 Birth mark (Mongolian blue spot). Certain races with darker skins, such as Asians, Africans and Chinese, can have birthmarks, mainly over the back and buttocks, which mimic bruising very closely. The shape of this birth mark – the Mongolian blue spot, is highly variable; sometimes, it is a large confluent area, in others, multiple small areas, as in this figure. The colour is dark blue, mimicking old, fading bruises which would also not be painful. These marks are present at birth, but can darken with age so becoming more noticeable. It is entirely harmless and tends to disappear during childhood.

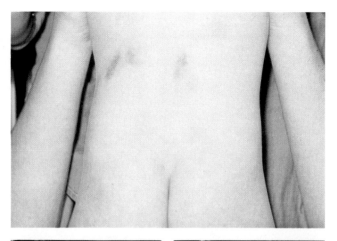

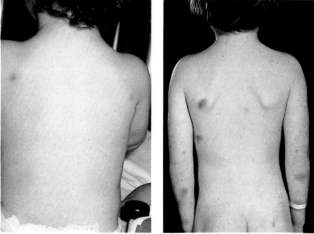

Fig. 29 Normal bruising on the back. The back, like the shins, is easily bruised during play or fighting. These three normal backs show varying degrees of bruising all acquired during the daily active life of the child. Backward falls in the toddler can easily cause bruising (bottom left), and as such falls tend to be repetitive, multiple bruises of different ages may be seen. In the active schoolchild many bruises can be acquired from falls from trees, fights, contact sports; the list is endless. Unless the bruising is extensive or recognisable (Fig. 39) then bruises on the back warrant little attention.

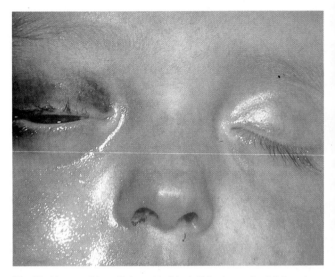

Fig. 30 Non-accidental injury. Accidental black eyes in childhood are common and result from many activities. However, black eyes in infants are far less common and rarely accidental, although a dropped object could cause such an injury. The child who has just acquired the skill of sitting alone has poorly developed saving reflexes, such as putting out an arm to correct leaning to one side. Even so, topples from the sitting position are unlikely to be forceful enough to cause a black eye. Thus in the very young, a traumatic black eye is generally the work of a third party. Again any number of people can be the perpetrator and a single incident may only be worth noting. However, repeated black eyes in the non-walking infant should be viewed with suspicion.

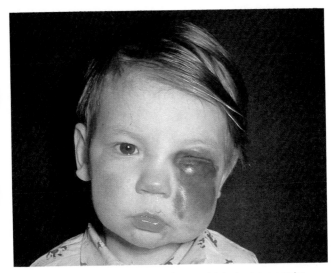

Fig. 31 Bleeding disorder. Yet again, any sinister bruising can be mimicked by a bleeding disorder. This young child has haemophilia and a slight blow to the eye caused this massive bleeding. The result is far worse than the injury in Fig. 30 and should, in theory, require far more force. The child with a mild bleeding tendency, who has not been diagnosed can, unfortunately, catch out the unwary observer, but, conversely, many parents claim when accused of NAI that their child bruises easily. This claim is usually false and can be easily checked by the hospital or primary care physician.

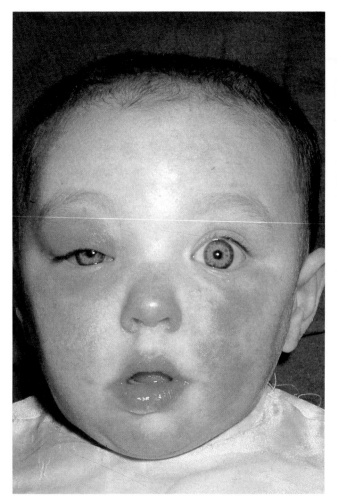

Fig. 32 Infection. The tissues around the eye are loose, even in an infant and this facilitates rapid spread of an infection through the tissues surrounding the eye, producing cellulitis. The eye itself is normally unaffected, but the surrounding tissues are swollen, hot and tender. The child is discomforted by the pain and will be fretful, but otherwise well. The picture mimics a recent black eye well, the area is tender, and the tissues are hot, discoloured and swollen. Such an appearance, resulting from infection can develop very rapidly, within a matter of hours and the parents will be totally unable to explain the appearance.

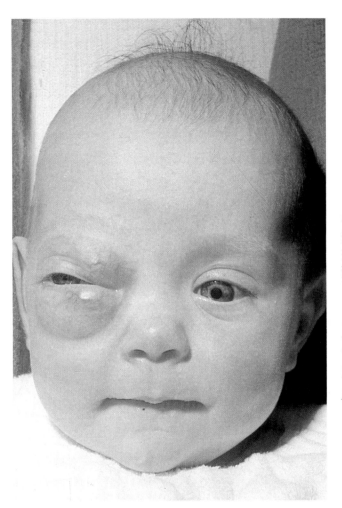

Fig. 33 Congenital abnormality. The most common blood vessel abnormality is the strawberry naevus (Figs. 11 and 21), but several other types exist (Fig. 13) which do not necessarily exhibit the brilliant strawberry colour. This child has an asymmetrical swelling around the eye caused by abnormal blood vessel formation. The overlying skin is faintly discoloured and reddened. A characteristic of naturally occurring, acquired abnormalities is that they are symmetrical (Fig. 88), however, congenital abnormalities may equally well be asymmetrical. The swelling in this child will not be tender nor painful and will remain constant, unlike the results of trauma.

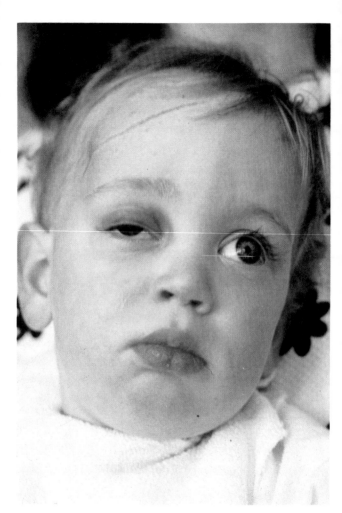

Fig. 34 Secondary cancer. This, fortunately is an extremely rare cause of a 'black eye', but, as it is so uncommon, could be mistaken for a traumatic black eye. The cancer causing the problem is usually deep in the body and may not have been detected before the changes in the eye occur. The bruising comes from pressure within the eye socket rather than from outside, so little swelling occurs initially. This child has a squint as a result of the secondary cancer; unless the child already has a squint, trauma is unlikely to cause such a problem. These figures of black eyes, of which only one is traumatic (Fig. 30), illustrate graphically how medical causes can mimic traumatic causes.

34

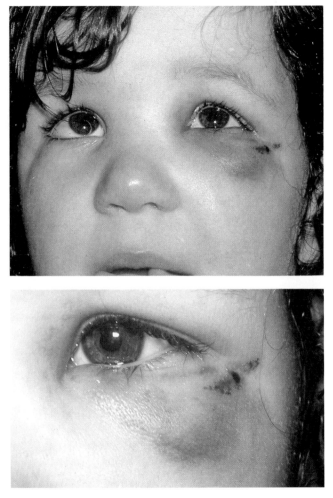

Fig. 35 Non-accidental injury. This child has an unpleasant black eye with an abrasion which may have been caused by a ring or a finger nail. There is, however, nothing about the injury shown which suggests that this is a deliberate injury by an adult, rather than accidental. This child has a pleading expression when confronted by an adult. This may be the reaction induced by repeated blows or may equally be fear of the camera. If assault is suspected, then injuries and the family circumstances should be checked. In this way, the injury can be said to be NAI, but it would be foolhardy to take action against the parents on this injury alone.

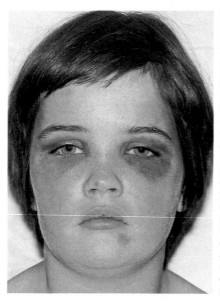

Fig. 36 Bilateral black eyes. Two black eyes are rarely accidental. They can occur with a fracture of the base of the skull, but this requires massive force, such as in a road traffic accident which would leave the child with other injuries. Assault is the most plausible explanation. Once this has been established, the perpetrator of the injury is less easy to determine. Sibling and playground rivalry are more dangerous than most parents.

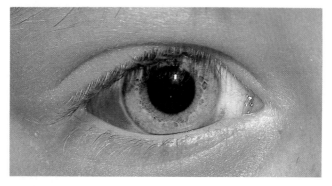

Fig. 37 Subconjunctival haemorrhage. Subconjunctival haemorrhage (see also Fig. 78) is bleeding between the cornea and the conjunctiva. Such bleeding requires force, but can occur naturally, for example during birth, or after a particularly violent coughing spasm, such as occurs in whooping cough. It may also result from a blow, either to the eye or surrounding tissues, however, this would be accompanied by bruising and swelling of these tissues. The haemorrhage may be induced by violent shaking of the child, or a blow to the head, distant from the eye. Whether accidental or deliberate, subconjunctival haemorrhage is the result of force and any explanation must include this.

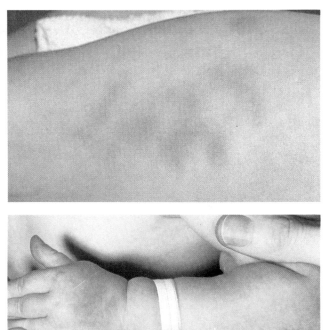

Fig. 38 Finger marks. Accidental bruising has no recognisable shape, the lesions have irregular outlines and, if multiple, are randomly placed, reflecting the random movements causing the damage. Recognisable marks or shapes on a child are more sinister. A child may fall against a sharp edge, such as a table, causing a bruise with straight edges, but finger marks are rarely accidental. Normal play does not cause obvious finger marks, even if quite violent such as throwing the child in the air or swinging him by the arms. Children are grasped between the fingers and thumb, so if finger marks are seen on the arm (top) the thumb mark should be sought on the other side of the arm. Placement of the observer's hand over the suspected markings allows a rough idea of the size of the damaging hand, which could be that of a child. The marks in the bottom picture are not so obviously finger marks, but the positioning of the bruises is curiously uniform, not a feature of accidental bruising, and finger tips fit well into this pattern. Such suspicion would be heightened if a corresponding thumb mark was found.

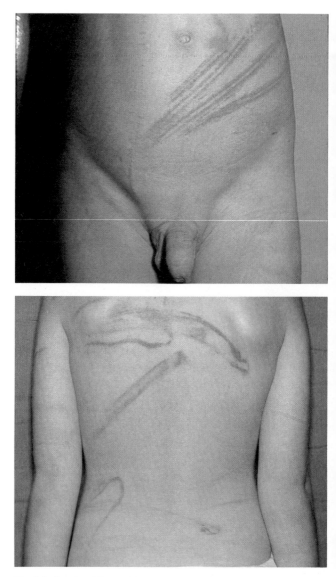

Fig. 39 Beating. These children bear evidence of obvious beating. The individual marks have straight lines, they are multiple, easily recognisable and could not have been self-inflicted. The child in the top picture has marks in an unusual site for a beating.

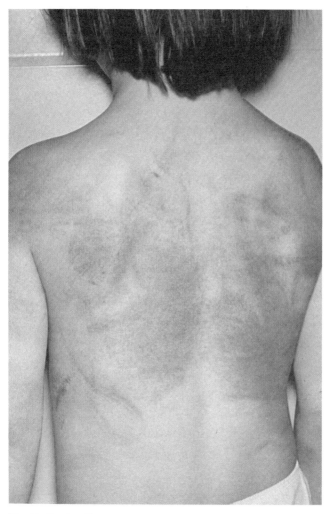

Fig. 40 Beating. The beating in this child is more extensive and the marks have merged. They are still recognisable marks of a deliberate beating. This child and the children in Fig. 39 have obviously been assaulted, but could it be justified? Until recently corporal punishment was condoned in the majority of our schools. Indeed physical pain has been an accepted means of correction for centuries. The children in Fig. 39 have received a few blows only but the child in this picture has been subjected to excessive violence. The question remains – is all beating unacceptable?

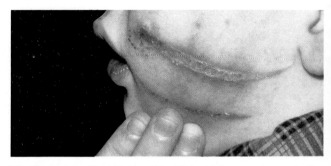

Fig. 41 Non-accidental injury. This child exhibits several aspects of NAI. He is young, although just walking and has two clearly definable marks on the face, both of which have straight edges. The lesions are infected which suggests that there has been a delay in seeking medical advice. On questioning, the explanation was readily forthcoming: two cuts from a riding crop, which were justified as necessary and acceptable corrective punishment. It is most difficult in these circumstances to decide on the correct course of action. If the family circumstances are stable and loving, albeit somewhat violent, should steps be taken to protect the child?

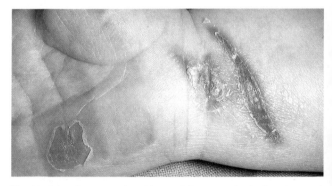

Fig. 42 Injury from restrainer. Young children restrict the freedom and social life of their parents considerably. Initially, regular and frequent feeding requires constant adult attendance and when the child can walk and, therefore, injure himself in limitless ways, adult surveillance is crucial. However, if the child is unable to move, less damage will occur. Infants rapidly learn how to escape from a cot, so restraining bands may be applied to the wrists and possibly ankles and anchored to the cot sides. The child becomes frantic with boredom, loss of familiar faces, but mainly from the feeling of restriction and struggles to free himself from the restrainers. Subsequently the restrainers are more firmly applied and can cause the illustrated injury. Although this injury is arguably not NAI, it does imply neglect.

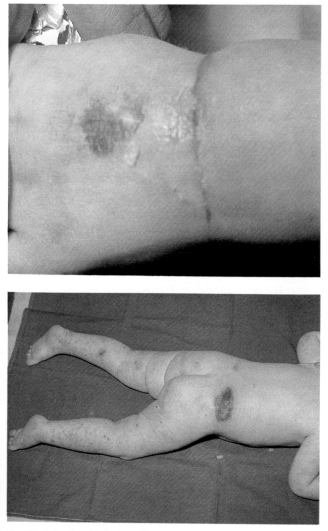

Fig. 43 Infective skin lesions. The lesion in the top picture has many similarities to the injury in Fig. 42. The lesion is a straight line, which could have been produced by a cord restrainer and there is damage to the back of the hand similar to that in Fig. 66. The similarity to NAI is seen even more vividly in the lower picture where the child has multiple bruises on the legs and back and an area of skin loss, on the flank, suggestive of a burn.

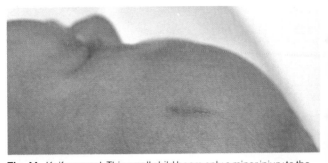

Fig. 44 Knife wound. This small child bears only a minor injury to the forehead. Initially this appears to be of little consequence, however, close inspection reveals a straight line injury without the surrounding swelling or bruising which would be expected if the child had fallen against a sharp edge, causing the damage. This injury was the result of a knife attack, which is highly worrying, even though the resultant damage is minor. The age of the child is of major relevance; the older child who can wield a knife, albeit haphazardly, can readily inflict such a wound on himself or his siblings.

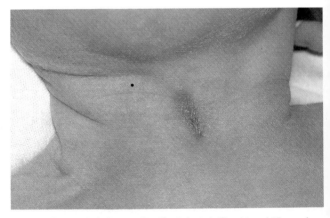

Fig. 45 Congenital abnormality. The infants in Fig. 44 and 45 are of approximately the same age and sport similar looking lesions. Both defects have straight line edges, and in neither is there bruising or swelling. The lesion in Fig. 45 is possibly more suspicious as it occurs on the neck – a normally protected area. It is however, a not uncommon congenital abnormality, which is frequently seen at the side of the neck, and results from failure of closure of developing channels. The defect would have been present at birth and, therefore, noted and documented, allowing rapid confirmation of the parents story.

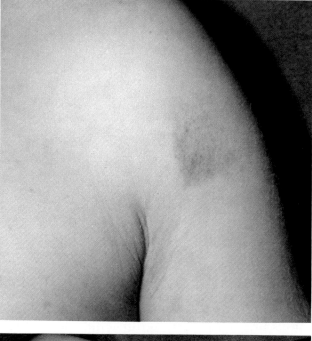

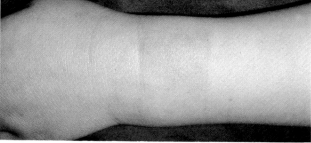

Fig. 46 Straight edged bruising. Neither of these injuries have immediately recognisable shapes, but both are well demarcated and have obvious straight line edges to them. The injury in the top picture is on an easily bruised part of the body and may have been caused by falling against a table corner, for example. The bruise in the lower picture bears similarities to the allergic reaction in Fig. 67. Thus both injuries have some characteristics of NAI, but both can also be explained accidentally. Care must be taken to unearth further suspicious problems, either physical or within the family fabric, before any action is taken.

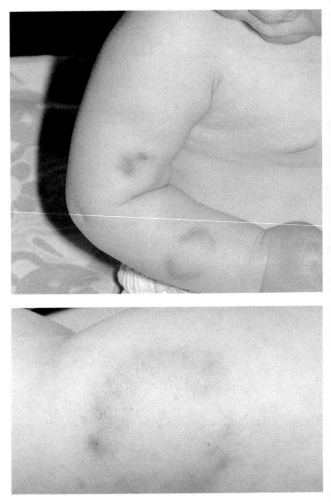

Fig. 47 Bites. Bites are common in childhood, normally inflicted by peers or siblings. Adult bites are unacceptable either as a means of relieving frustration or as a means of correction. Bite marks are usually distinctive: a circle consisting of two discontinuous semi-circles corresponding to the upper and lower teeth. If the perpetrator has abnormal dentition, such as loss of several teeth, the bite mark would reflect this. There is no central bruising, although there may be generalised swelling of the area. The size and shape of the bite is of prime importance. Children bite each other avidly and also seem to delight in tormenting the family pet, with predictable results (Fig. 48).

44

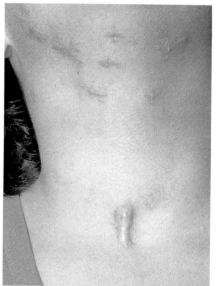

Fig. 48 Dog bite. This older girl displays the healing scars of a dog bite on her neck. The difference in the shape of the bite from human bites (Fig. 47) can easily be seen, despite the lack of bruising and swelling of the acute injury. This was the result of a bite from a large dog; bites of smaller dogs or cats with a more circular bite may be more difficult to differentiate. More exotic pets are now being kept in the home and there may be little difference in human and monkey bites!

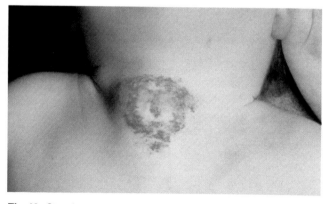

Fig. 49 Strawberry naevus. This strawberry naevus demonstrates clearly the mode of resolution of this congenital malformation. Initially the centre of the naevus resolves leaving a circular lesion, reminiscent of a bite mark. However, the circle is continuous and is not tender. The naevus will be raised, but have small irregularities in its surface, like a strawberry; the swelling after a bite is tender and uniform with no irregularities.

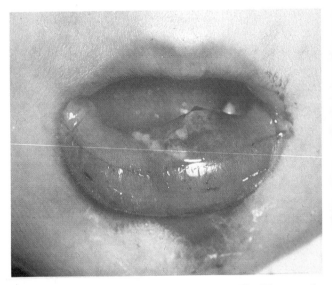

Fig. 50 Injury to mouth. Damage to the mouth (see Fig. 85) can easily occur accidentally from collisions or falls in the toddler. The older, more stable child is less likely to injure the mouth, as saving reflexes cause him to break his fall with his arms. A deliberate blow to the mouth will cause swelling of the lips and damage to the inner surface of the lip as it is forced against the teeth. In the infant, a feeding bottle may be rammed into the mouth in a desperate attempt to quieten the infant. If the teat catches under the tongue, the frenulum of the tongue may be torn, and the frenulum of the upper lip may be damaged by the bottle rim. Damage to the lips in an older child is more likely to result from a blow by the fist. If damage to the lips is seen, the inside of the mouth should be inspected to reveal the extent of the injury.

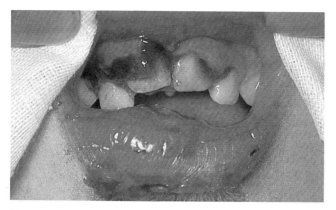

Fig. 51 Deranged teeth. Considerable force is required to displace teeth. The child who falls over, hitting his mouth on a solid surface usually chips the tooth rather than displacing it. If such damage is found, the explanation must include violence. A blow to the mouth might conceivably cause this damage, but it is more likely to have resulted from a solid object being forced up into the mouth. A child subjected to an assault of such force should be protected as rapidly as possible.

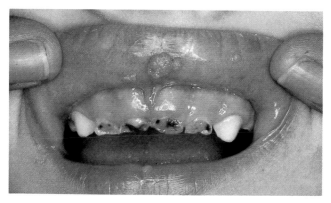

Fig. 52 Dental caries. These teeth have been slowly destroyed by dental caries, the so called 'milk teeth syndrome'. This is caused by the infant having a bottle of milk or sweet juice constantly in its mouth day and night. The teeth are continually bathed in sugary liquid which facilitates decay by caries. This could be a sign of over zealous mothering or a sign of neglect, where the child is left in the cot with a bottle to comfort it and otherwise neglected. The latter situation is more likely if the child is noted to be slow in development, especially of speech, which could be a sign of poor stimulation.

Burns

Technology, together with the need to cook and heat, has produced a home environment fraught with danger to the young child. Both major and minor accidental burns are distressingly common in infants and toddlers. Parental carelessness or forgetfulness increase the risk to the young child, and the desire to learn by imitation may have unpleasant consequences. The common habit of testing the temperature of the iron with a light touch may be harm-free to an adult, but may cause a significant burn in the child. Burns and scalds which are deliberately inflicted can, therefore, be extremely difficult to differentiate from those caused accidentally. It is important, therefore, to take into account all aspects of the case, including social conditions and treatment of the siblings as well as the explanation. A burn may have been accidental, but if not the first to the child or within the family, there may be an element of neglect. If the circumstances are thought to be suspicious, it is important to examine the child for any other injuries. Almost half of the children deliberately burnt have suffered a previous non-accidental fracture.

Certain injuries are immediately alerting, for example, scalds to the feet and buttocks (Fig. 53) caused by forcing the child into scalding water. A similar lesion to Fig. 53, with an identical distribution is caused by an inherited skin disease (Fig. 54) and other diseases (Figs. 56 and 57) which resemble burns or healing scars, similarly occur naturally.

Major burns can be accidental; Fig. 60 shows the effect of a burst hot water bottle. Note specifically the irregular outline to the injury, also a feature of the lesions shown in Fig. 61 and 62. An irregular outline favours a natural or accidental aetiology. Conversely, straight lines demarcating part of the injury (Figs. 63 and 64) argue strongly in favour of a non-accidental cause.

The shape of the injury is important; does it resemble any household object? Deliberate branding (Fig. 65) produces a regular outline, seen also in Fig. 66 from a naturally occurring disease. However, the sharply demarcated lesion in Fig. 67 is, in fact, an allergy to a cheap bangle watch. Multiple lesions (Figs. 68 and 69) are also immediately alerting. Even a small child will jump back once he is burnt and will not return for a second dose. However, the two burns seen in Fig. 70 were caused by a child grabbing the electric fire element and catching her wrist on the hot guard bars.

The mechanism of burning is of interest. Friction burns (Fig. 69) may be common on the buttocks or stomach and chest, if the child is sliding downhill on a rough surface during play, but multiple friction burns in non-pressure areas should be viewed with suspicion.

A common burning object, readily to hand at moments of stress or anger, is a cigarette. Cigarette burns (Fig. 71) are recognisable by their shape: a small, well circumscribed, circular lesion. Frequently cigarette burns are multiple. However, the lesions shown in Figs. 72-74 demonstrate all these characteristics and are all naturally occurring.

Non-accidental burns to the mouth are not common, but may be produced by holding a hot object, such as an iron, to the lips. More commonly, oral burns are caused by domestic caustic substances (Fig. 75) such as caustic soda. Even if the burn is caused by scalding water placed against the lips, it is unlikely that the child would drink, so that burns in the mouth are more suggestive of accidental voluntary ingestion.

Certain cultures use heat to kill the 'evil spirits' causing the illness and children may sport extensive scarring (Fig. 77) from well-meant, but inappropriate medicinal treatment.

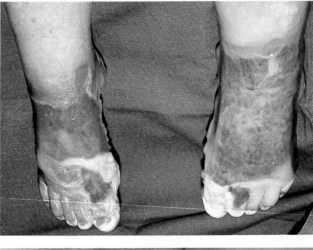

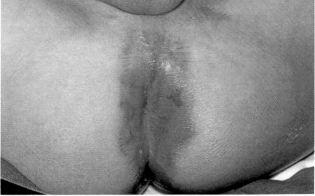

Fig. 53 Scalds from bath. Sadly this is not an uncommon injury. The parent becomes exasperated by a day of childhood provocation and fills the nightly bath with hotter water than normal. The child is then grabbed, usually around the chest, and dumped unceremoniously into the water. The feet suffer most as they enter the water first and the child then struggles to keep the rest of his body out of the water. If forced downwards, the legs flex and are, therefore, spared, but the buttocks are scalded. The extent of the burn depends on the amount of the body immersed and for what length of time. The distribution shown here – scalded buttocks and feet, the feet more severely affected, is the most common distribution. The child will be struggling violently so may have splash marks elsewhere on his body, as indeed may the perpetrator.

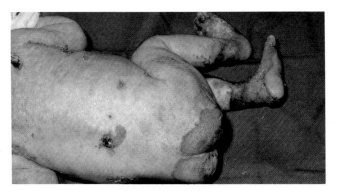

Fig. 54 Inherited skin disease. The child exhibits skin damage in the same distribution as Fig. 53, with some 'splash' marks on the trunk. However, careful examination reveals that part of the soles of the feet are spared whilst the legs are affected to above the ankle, an unlikely distribution if the damage was caused by the feet being thrust into scalding water. Also the 'splash' lesions are at different stages of healing; some look new, others have scar formation, making immersion unlikely unless repeated. This is an uncommon skin disease, but is inherited so siblings may be similarly affected, arousing suspicions.

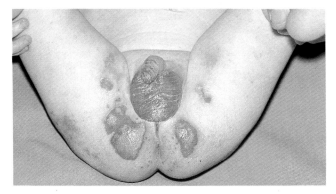

Fig. 55 Burn to buttocks. An alternative to dunking the child in a scalding bath is to sit him on a hot surface; this may be the oven hot plate, or radiator or the top of a boiler. The areas of the buttocks supporting most pressure, which depends partly on the position of the child, will be most affected. If the child has flexed his hips upwards, only the buttocks will be burnt, with sparing of the skin in the natal cleft. If the legs are relaxed then the burn would extend over more of the buttock and onto the posterior region of the thigh. In the male, the scrotum may also be affected.

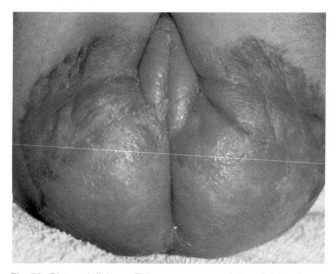

Fig. 56 Dietary deficiency. This appearance could be mistaken for a healing scald; it is certainly of the right distribution. However, there is no plane of separation between normal skin and eschar tissue which would be expected after a burn, and it is not the correct colour for healed scar tissue. As the child is forced into the water, he may keep his legs together which would have the effect of sparing the skin folds in the groin. There is no such sparing in this illustration. It is unlikely that the child would be gently lowered into the water in non-accidental scaldings, they are usually grabbed and dumped feet first. An isolated scald on the buttock is, therefore, less likely to be non-accidental.

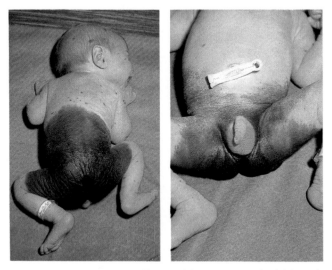

Fig. 57 Extensive birth mark. This child shows an extensive birth mark (mole) covering the buttocks, thighs and trunk. The simple expedient of turning the infant over reveals that vital parts of the anatomy have been spared, which would be impossible if the cause had been a burn or a scald. This demonstrates simply, but graphically, the need to search for other evidence about the child in an attempt to confirm or allay fears of non-accidental injury, before taking any further action.

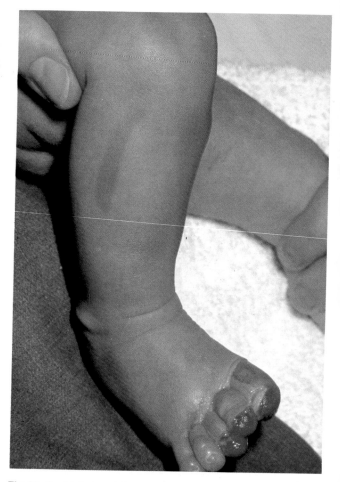

Fig. 58 Scalds to toes. Infants are not immune from being immersed in scalding water. However, infant skin is less resistant to heat than adult skin and scalds occur at lower temperatures. Hence, such a small scald, affecting the toes only, may happen accidentally. If one parent fills the bath without testing the temperature, assuming that the other will, the first part of the infant to test the scalding water may be the foot. The child is withdrawn at the first scream so the extent of lesion is small. Such an injury may convince the investigator that the cause was accidental. However, great pain is suffered by the infant from such damage, and the more devious of abusers may inflict minor, non-suspicious injuries deliberately.

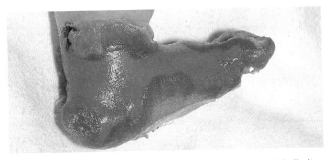

Fig. 59 Inherited skin disease. This demonstrates the great similarity to a scalded infant foot. There is an obvious line of demarcation, skin loss over the foot and a similar inflamed appearance to that in Fig. 53 (top). This is caused by the same inherited disease shown in Fig. 54, it is probable, therefore, that other areas of the body will be affected. However, this does illustrate well the difficulty that may be encountered if such a problem is taken in isolation. The importance of approaching such a dilemma from every angle, physical, psychological and social, cannot be overstressed.

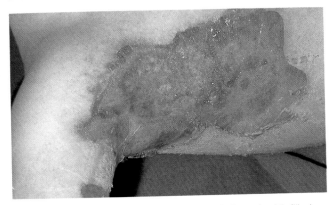

Fig. 60 Scald. This unpleasant scald occurred when a freshly filled hot water bottle burst. The scald has no recognisable shape and has an irregular edge, suggesting that an accidental injury is the most probable explanation. There are also scalds on the arm, possibly where the child was hugging the bottle. If the scald had been deliberate, the arm would probably have been spared as the child tried to keep other parts of his body away from the pain. If the arm had been intentionally forced down onto a hot object, finger mark bruising would be apparent. The explanation, therefore, fits both major and minor elements of the injury.

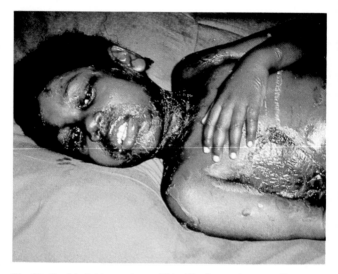

Fig. 61 Scalded skin syndrome. This skin disease is caused by a virulent and contagious bacterium and the skin changes mimic scalding closely, as suggested by its common name. The disease has, therefore, been the cause of many unwarranted accusations. This illustration is of the gross form where much of the skin all over the body has been affected. Differentiation between infection and burn will not be difficult as the child will not be in pain, but will be acutely ill. A superficial burn of such magnitude would be unbearably painful but otherwise the child would be alert and well. Smaller lesions can cause great problems in differentiation. Skin loss occurs rapidly as the infection spreads under the skin, so it is conceivable that the child may be put to bed looking normal, and awake with a scald-like lesion, with no explanation forthcoming from the parents. Aspects to consider are:– (i) pain, a superficial burn is highly painful, scalded skin syndrome is not, (ii) shape, if the cause is infection the shape is irregular, a non-accidental scald may have a regular outline, (iii) any other marks, such as bruises or cuts which would argue in favour of deliberate assault.

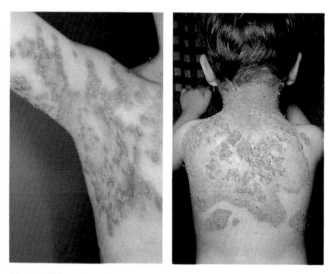

Fig. 62 Skin rashes. At first glance, both of these skin rashes could be mistaken for burns or scalds. A burn at the site of the rash on the left could have resulted from a child pulling down a saucepan from the stove. It is difficult to conceive of a self-inflicted injury in the location on the right, but again accidental spillage by a third person is possible. Both rashes show irregular outlines, more in keeping with accidental or naturally-occurring causes. The child on the left shows a blistering skin rash with the blisters at different stages of healing, more evidence against a scald or burn which would have occurred at one time only. The child on the right demonstrates the result of contact allergy, possibly against clothing dyes or detergent or hair shampoo. Such an allergy may be severe, causing blistering and disruption of the superficial skin. Healing would be uniform, unlike that on the left. Unlike a burn which would be intensely painful, this rash may be unbearably itchy.

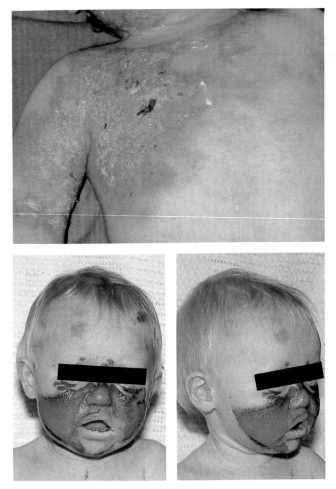

Fig. 63 Deliberate burns. The burns illustrated in these figures have all been deliberately inflicted. The most striking aspect they have in common is a straight margin to the burn. This is seen on the chest, away from the affected arm in the top picture and seen very strikingly on the face in the lower figure. Such burns are compatible with a cloth dipped in scalding water, being placed or slapped across the child's body. In the top picture, possibly a tea-towel was used, with the edge falling on the chest. In the lower picture, a corner of a face cloth may have caused the well-defined edges. Further evidence suggestive of assault can be seen in this child: bruising and an abrasion occurring on the forehead are approximately of the same age as the scald.

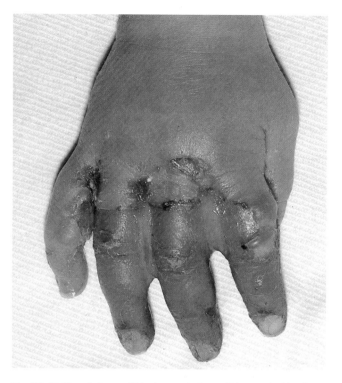

Fig. 64 Deliberate burns. This demonstrates well the result of forcing the hand into scalding water. Three of the fingers are affected and again there is a straight line rigidly demarcating the normal and affected skin. The scalds on the little finger and back of the hand were probably caused by splashing as the child struggled. The lesions in this picture and Fig. 63 are identical to those caused by the scalded skin syndrome (vide supra) with raw skin and pus formation. The main argument against such a cause is the regular outline and potentially recognisable shape of the burn.

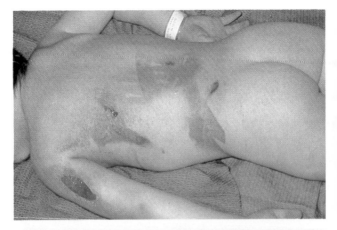

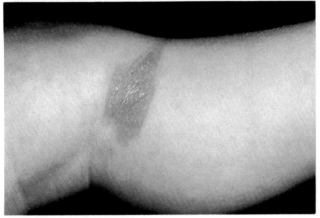

Fig. 65 Deliberate branding. There can be little doubt that this child has been subjected to a non-accidental assault. He has multiple abrasions and burn marks on his back and arm (top) and leg (bottom). The mark on his arm and just above the buttock on the same side bear several characteristics of deliberate injury. Multiple marks of this nature are unlikely to have been caused accidentally; the brand marks have well demarcated edges and all areas of damage are of a similar age, suggesting a single incident. It is difficult to conceive of a single instrument causing all the marks on this child, but the lesion on the arm is sufficiently sinister to cause a high degree of concern. Immediate steps must be taken to safeguard this child and admission to hospital is frequently the easiest method of achieving this. Parents generally accept such an admission, despite the anxiety and guilt caused by their actions.

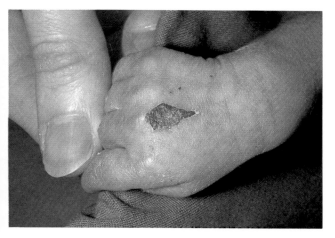

Fig. 66 Inherited skin disease. This infant suffers from a mild variant of the disease shown in Figs. 54 and 59. Skin damage in this disease is not extensive, heals without scarring and may occur either as single or multiple lesions. The problem illustrated has several suspicious aspects. The child is young and immobile and, therefore, unlikely to have caused the lesion himself; it is a well demarcated area with straight edges and, if this is the first presentation, there will be no convincing explanation forthcoming. If there were multiple such lesions, all without explanation, suspicions would be heightened further. This demonstrates the degree of difficulty faced when attempting to elucidate the cause of problems in the immobile child, who should be injury-free. The immobile group of children also includes the severely handicapped, who are also more at risk of battering.

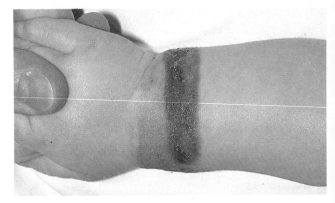

Fig. 67   Allergy. This mark was caused by an allergy to a cheap bangle watch. The watch had been a gift several months previously and, as the child had grown, so the bangle became tighter causing sweating under the watch. The child eventually became allergic to the nickel in the bangle, producing the illustrated lesion. However, again there are several features which could rouse suspicion. The area is well-demarcated with straight line margins. A possible non-accidental cause would be the tight application of restrainers, where the child is tied in an outstretched position and the subsequent struggling causes a friction burn, the slight lateral movement causing the reddened area either side. This again highlights difficulties for the would-be accuser, especially as allergy does not necessarily occur immediately and may appear after months or years of contact with the article to which the person then becomes allergic.

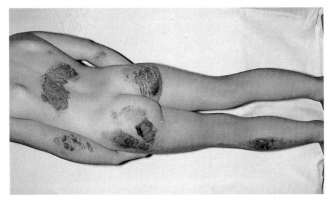

Fig. 68 Multiple burns. There are no regular outlines to these burns, but as there are many areas of damage, all at similar stages of healing, grave doubts as to their cause must be entertained. Such widespread afflictions suggest that the child is in considerable danger and should be removed from the environment immediately. This child was deliberately tied to a car by one leg and dragged along the ground for some distance. When such damage to a child is encountered, it is probably safer to err on the side of caution, unless a totally plausible and corroborated explanation is forthcoming. The child should be hospitalised immediately, therefore circumventing the necessity of immediate accusation, whilst protecting the child and allowing the situation to be assessed.

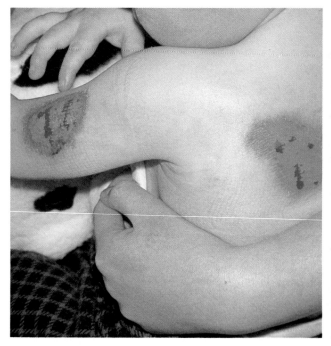

Fig. 69 Friction burns. Friction burns are relatively common in children. There is a fascination for sliding down playground slides, but if these are not available, invention supervenes. The child may slide down a slope on a board and sustain friction burns at the inevitable unhorsing, or if such artefacts are not available, just slide down in his clothes. The burns would, therefore, be over pressure points such as the buttocks or hips and chest and possibly hands. Friction burns are less likely to occur over non pressure-bearing areas such as the upper arm, as there is no solid surface to rub against. It is difficult to understand, therefore, how the two burns shown here could have been self-inflicted or happened accidentally. A plausible explanation must be elicited.

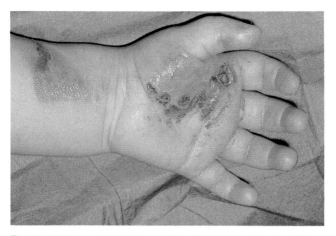

Fig. 70 Multiple accidental burns. This child who is only just mobile displays suspicious burns. They are multiple and the burn on the wrist has a straight edge. They were caused by the inquisitive crawler putting her hand between the protective bars of an electric fire and grasping the element. The wrist was caught as she withdrew her hand rapidly. This is a most plausible explanation. It is impossible to know, however, whether the child placed her hand on the element voluntarily or was forced to do so. Possibly the only way to determine would be to delve deeper into social circumstances and increase surveillance. It is in these cases that innocent parents may become indignant and embarrassed. There may be very little data on which to base an acceptance or rejection of the parents' explanation. To reject may cause considerable family disruption, to accept, may, in the extreme, kill the child.

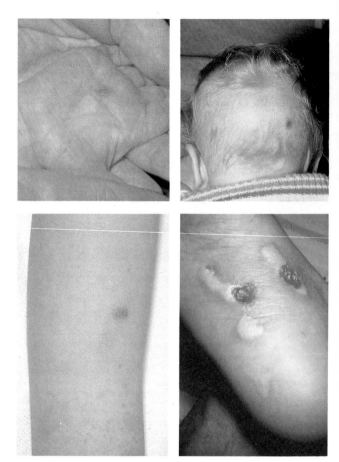

Fig. 71 Cigarette burns. Cigarette burns are a common non-accidental injury. The rush of anger or resentment, coupled with a desire to hurt or punish, is easily satisfied by stubbing out a cigarette on the child. The injury is painful and has the desired effect of distressing the child, but is a minor injury with no serious complications and can be easily explained to the casual observer. Healing is rapid so medical attention and, therefore, surveillance, is not required. Cigarette burns occur at any age, on all parts of the body. Those to the head (top right) may not be visible under covering hair. The result of all cigarette burns is a small, circular, punched-out area of skin loss (top left). Single cigarette burns are virtually impossible to diagnose unless the situation is already worrying, but multiple punched out lesions, (bottom right) should lead more readily to the correct conclusion.

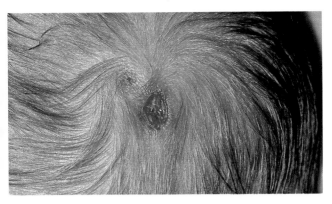

Fig. 72 Congenital skin defect. This and the following two illustrations demonstrate the dangers of reaching sinister conclusions on either single or multiple round lesions. This scalp defect is virtually identical to a cigarette burn: circular, well demarcated with loss of superficial skin. The surrounding hair may well have covered the area, and so, when suddenly seen may be misinterpreted, especially as the damage looks fresh. Unlike skin diseases or rashes, this defect may be single, thus depriving the observer of other helpful guiding aids.

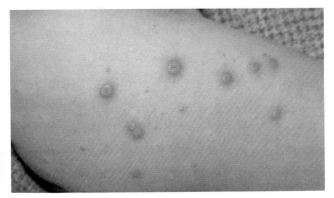

Fig. 73 Skin rash. This rash is common in childhood, although, this specific variant occurs less frequently. It may accompany many childhood infections, whether bacterial, viral or fungal and may result from drug therapy with a large number of different drugs. Initially, the child may be thought to be a victim of multiple quick touches with a lighted cigarette, producing blisters. The other smaller spots in-between could conceivably have been caused by flicked ash. Careful observation and precise self-questioning as to whether such appearances are compatible with a sinister interpretation are required before further action is taken.

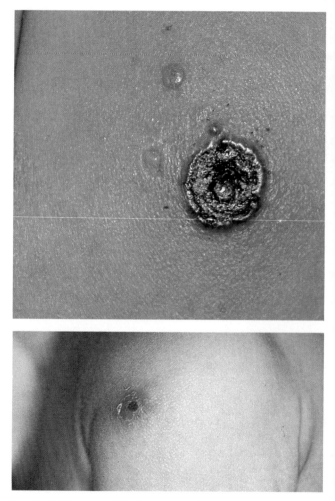

Fig. 74 B.C.G. scars. B.C.G. vaccination is usually administered to secondary school children. There are, however, indications for giving the younger child or infant the vaccination, for example, if the family is in contact with tuberculosis. Indeed, one area in Britain has only recently stopped giving B.C.G. to all babies at birth. The reaction to B.C.G. varies enormously from a minor red flare to an ulcer or abscess as shown here. If the child is given B.C.G. at an age other than normal, such small round punched out lesions may be viewed with suspicion. These B.C.G. reactions also tend to be painful, in keeping with a superficial burn.

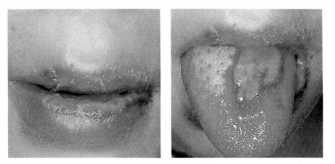

Fig. 75 Caustic burn. This child's lips are affected on the internal surfaces. Deliberate burns to the mouth would affect the outer surfaces, possibly with damage to the surrounding skin. If a cup of scalding water was placed against the lips, the immediate reaction of pursing the lips would similarly cause damage to the outer aspects of the lips. It is highly unlikely that the child could be forced to take any of the scalding liquid into the mouth (right) so the most likely explanation would be that the child drank voluntarily. The next question to be asked, however, is whether the caustic fluid was left around deliberately for the child or whether there was an element of neglect in allowing the child access to such material.

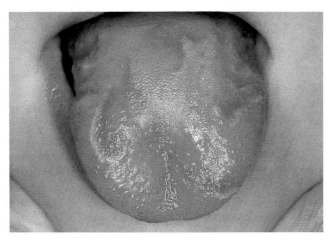

Fig. 76 Geographical tongue. This abnormality of the tongue: loss of taste-bud bearing skin, is quite common. It is entirely harmless, but bears similarities to the caustic burn (Fig. 75). The child is unlikely, however, to have extensive scalding to the tongue without some damage to the lips. Also the geographical tongue is painless, whereas a burnt mouth or tongue is extremely painful.

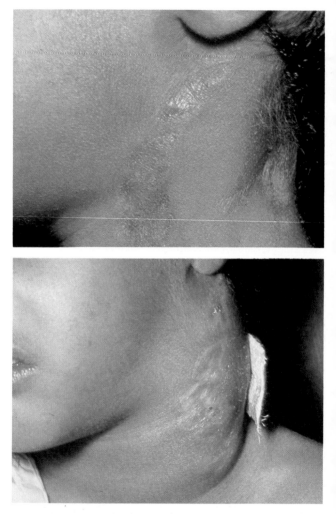

Fig. 77 Scars of healing. Certain cultures still depend heavily on the local 'medicine man'. The methods of healing used by such a person are highly varied and sometimes dangerous; one such is the use of heat. Heat is thought to kill the evil spirit causing the disease. If there is an obvious abnormality, heat is applied directly to that area, as in these cases, but if there is a general illness, quite extensive burnings are used. If the disease resolves with time, all is well; if not, the child may be subjected to further treatments and may become extensively burnt and scarred.

External Markers of Internal Injury

Many children subjected to physical abuse display obvious signs of their injuries. However, in some children, severe internal damage can be produced with little or no external evidence, and in such cases it is difficult to distinguish between deliberate and accidental injury. Since some medical conditions can resemble non-accidental injury, it is important not to view any suspected injury in isolation from the medical history of the child and family circumstances.

Head injuries have the most serious consequences, and are a frequent cause of death in abused children. Bleeding from the ear may be the result of fracture of the base of the skull, or may simply be caused by injury to the ear itself. Subconjunctival haemorrhage (Fig. 78) may result from a minor blow to the eye, from a severe injury to the head (caused for instance by shaking the child) which results in intracranial haemorrhage, or may only be the result of coughing, especially in whooping cough. In cases of intracranial injury there may be immediate and obvious symptoms such as convulsions and vomiting; although if there is a slow accumulation of blood (a subdural haemorrhage, Fig. 79) there may be subtle changes in the level of consciousness or personality, which are much harder to recognise if contact with the child is intermittent.

Fractures of the skull of an infant require comparatively little force. There may be bleeding into the scalp (Fig. 80) which raises a bump and feels soft and boggy.

Accidental fractures of the long bones are rare in children under one year old, but may occur accidentally as a result of excessive twisting or pulling when changing a nappy. Fractures of the ends of the long bones, usually caused by violent pulling, rarely produce obvious external signs. Behavioural change may be the only indicator, such as in the toddler who suddenly refuses to walk, or who screams when being dressed or when one limb is touched.

Broken ribs, caused by violent shaking or blows, may also be difficult to detect in a small child, and a careful search should be made for other signs of injury such as grip marks or bruises before the child is referred for X-ray or Scan, since it is clearly dangerous and impracticable to

X-ray and/or Scan very small children as a matter of routine.

Even in the presence of an obvious fracture, medical conditions predisposing to easy fractures such as osteogenesis imperfecta (brittle bone disease) or spina bifida, or the use of steroids, must be excluded before a diagnosis of non-accidental injury can be made.

Fractured ribs heal with callous formation which may be visible in a thin child. It should be remembered though, that these can resemble the 'rosary' of rickets (Fig. 81). Rickets itself may not be the result of neglect either, but may be caused by a metabolic deficiency.

A swelling around the eye may be caused by bleeding following trauma, or may be the result of infection. In coloured children differentiation may be difficult (Fig. 83). One common pointer to excessive force in such a situation are 'grip marks' on both sides of the face. A swelling of the cheek (Fig. 84) may be a fracture but may also be due to mumps, infection or a tumour.

Minor trauma around the mouth (Fig. 85) warrants closer inspection. Injuries such as this may be accidental or congenital, (Fig. 86), but if accompanied by a torn frenulum of the tongue or upper lip, or deranged teeth, a more suspicious approach may be justified since injuries like these are frequently the result of a 'feeding-battle'.

As a general rule any abnormality which is bilateral and symmetrical is caused by disease rather than injury.

Examples of such defects are those caused by severe asthma (Fig. 82), inherited problems (Fig. 87) or following polio (Fig. 88). Unilateral abnormalities should be regarded with more suspicion, although many will have a medical cause. Fig. 89 shows rickets of the legs, whereas Fig. 90 is a fracture of the tibia. Fractures may cause asymmetry or swelling from deep bleeding, but swelling may also be caused by tumours (Fig. 91 left), or bony infection, such as osteomyelitis (Fig. 92), or muscle disease (Fig. 91 right). Swellings in infants are less likely to be caused by self-injury, because of the force required. Fig. 93 shows swelling resulting from assault whilst Fig. 94 was caused by birth injury and Fig. 95 by a tumour.

Deliberate injury causing damage to internal organs such as the liver, spleen or kidneys would require great force such as that from a punch or a kick. This type of injury is rare and is almost always the result of assault. However, as in all cases, it is vital to exclude medical causes before a more sinister interpretation of a disorder is considered.

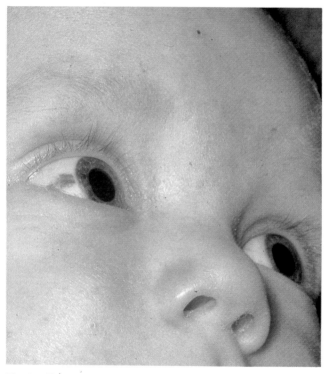

Fig. 78   Subconjunctival haemorrhage. This child has a small subconjunctival haemorrhage; the bleeding may, however, be extensive and extend behind the visible eye, but does not cover the iris or pupil. Spontaneous subconjunctival haemorrhages are rare in normal healthy children as some degree of violence is required. Haemorrhage may occur during birth or an attack of whooping cough but usually clears within two weeks. Other causes include a direct blow to the eye or the bony surround, either by a fist, for example, or the mobile infant colliding or falling against a hard object. Alternatively, it may result from a blow to the skull remote from the eye, or with severe intracranial bleeding. A small haemorrhage, such as this, in isolation does not warrant suspicion unless accompanied by other unexplained minor injuries or a known family history of violence.

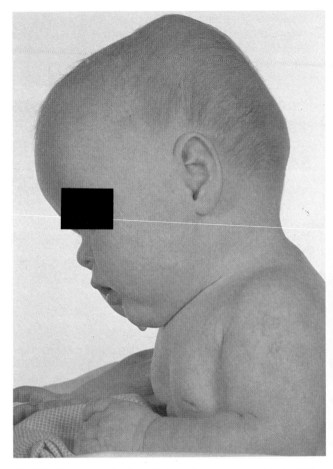

Fig. 79 Subdural collections. Subdural haemorrhages are caused by damage to the veins which pass from the brain to the major venous system in the head. Damage is caused when the brain moves relative to the skull causing tearing of the small veins. This only occurs with violence such as a car crash or fall onto the head. It may also happen if the child is violently shaken and the head jerked back and forth rapidly. If the bleeding is brisk the child may start fitting or lose consciousness. If, however, there is only a gradual ooze, pressure slowly increases in the head. Such pressure may cause changes in personality or consciousness some time after the assault. In the infant, before the skull bones have fused, the collections may become large enough to change the shape of the head, as in this child. The presence of the collection is always alarming and the cause must be sought.

74

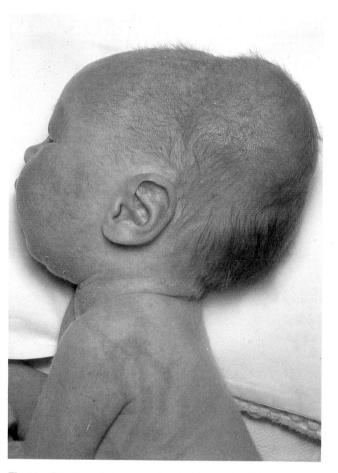

Fig. 80   Bleeding into the scalp. The skull bones of an infant are soft and pliable so do not tend to fracture easily. Nevertheless, the amount of force required to produce a fracture of the infant skull is quite small. There may be no external signs apart from irritability, but bleeding may occur into the scalp, either from the bone edges or from damaged scalp vessels. This produces a swelling under the scalp as seen here. Unlike the deformities in Fig.79, which are hard, this will have a soft, boggy feeling. This particular haemorrhage was caused at birth and is larger than most resulting from underlying fractures. However, blood is only slowly absorbed so the boggy sensation may persist for several months, possibly trapping the enthusiastic, but unwary observer into making false assumptions.

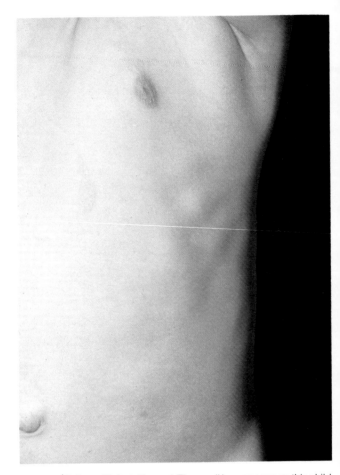

Fig. 81 Rickets. 'Rickety Rosary'. The small bumps seen on this child are caused by expansion of the bone ends, which occurs during rickets. When a bone is broken, the broken ends become covered by excess new bone, called callous, which is gradually remodelled to return the bone to its original shape. This callous formation over broken ribs may be seen as similar bumps in a thin child. The lumps shown here are symmetrical i.e. they occur at the same place on each rib, which would be unlikely if the ribs had been fractured accidentally or non-accidentally. Rib fractures are seen in babies whose chest has been squeezed during violent shaking and multiple ribs may have been fractured. Rickets also causes swelling of the ends of the long bones, seen as swollen ankles and wrists; such a symmetrical distribution would make non-accidental injury unlikely.

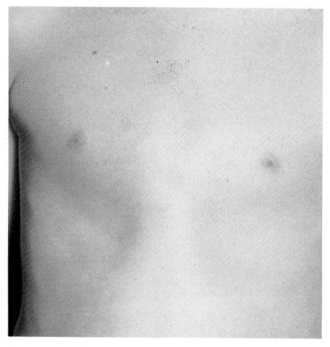

Fig. 82   Chest deformity. The deformity shown in this child is
symmetrical and is a common complication of severe asthma. It is
caused by overaction of the diaphragm during a wheezy period, which
tends to pull the soft childhood ribs inwards. Eventually, this deformity
becomes fixed, but old photographs will not show any chest problem.
It would be difficult to think of a non-accidental mechanism by which
these deformities would have been caused, and also maintained in a
growing child, in whom active remodelling occurs in order to return any
defect to the status quo.

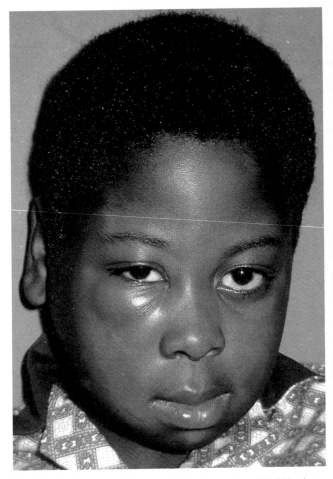

Fig.83   Swelling around the eye. Bruising in a coloured child is often
very difficult to detect. The swelling beneath this child's eye may be
due to bruising, a bleeding disorder, or infection. If infection was the
cause, the swelling would be hot and tender; however, after injury, if
the blood was under pressure or overlying a fracture, the swelling
might also be hot and tender. A blow to the eye, producing a 'black
eye' usually causes swelling both above and below the eye, so if
violence is considered, an injury must be postulated that would cause
such a localised swelling. The deformity is unilateral making a
generalised disease less likely, but not impossible; again care must be
exercised before accusations are levelled.

78

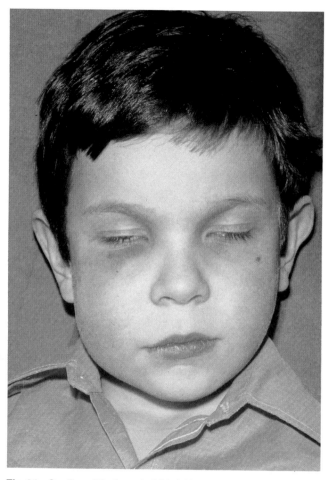

Fig. 84 Swelling of the face. A child of this age may present with a swelling of the side of the face for several reasons. Mumps is common in young school children and may affect one side only; a dental abscess will also cause one-sided swelling and in both instances the swelling will be tender. Playground disagreements are frequently settled physically and the resultant swelling may be large, especially if weapons, such as satchels, have been used. Infection of the muscle will cause a considerable bulge, as will a tumour of the bone, which will not be tender. The face is injured frequently, either during fighting or play in the mobile child, and bruises or bumps often have the same significance as bruising on the legs.

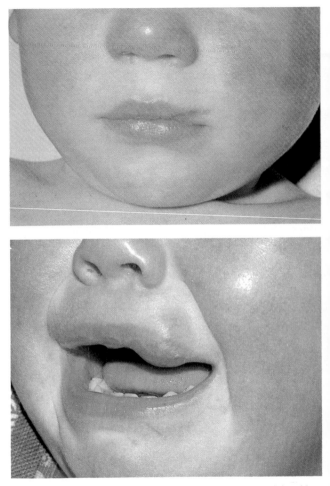

Fig. 85   Trauma of lips. The young, mobile child is prone to injure his head, as many solid household objects are at the head-height of an enthusiastic, but inexperienced toddler. Although not a common site of injury, bruises and cuts around the mouth are easily caused accidentally. This is not so in the immobile child. Also, damage to the mouth, such as tearing of the frenulum of the lower lip or tongue, or disruption of the teeth, implies major violence, such as a feeding bottle being rammed into the mouth. It is of great importance, therefore, to look in the child's mouth as a minor lip injury may overlay mouth trauma. Obviously a normal mouth will not exclude non-accidental injury, but a damaged one may heighten suspicion.

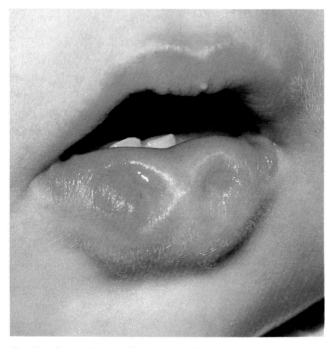

Fig. 86   Congenital pits of the lower lip. These pits are congenital deformities of the lower lip, but look as though they might have been caused by repeated trauma, such as forcing the lip against the teeth, so producing lacerations. Although the child would have been born with a defect of the lower lip, congenital malformations are not static and can change with the growth of the child, so such defects may not necessarily be obvious in old photographs, if these are being used to check whether abnormalities are new or old. Another check for naturally-occurring defects of the lips is to look at the ears. Lips and ears are linked during development, so if changes are present in both, any sinister interpretation is unlikely.

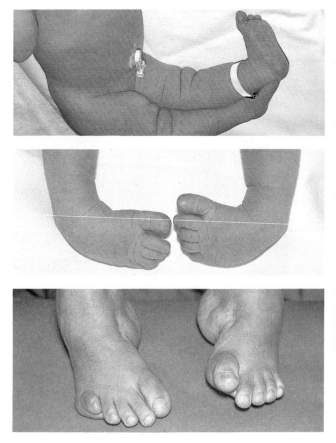

Fig. 87 Congenital deformities. The deformities shown in these figures are all symmetrical, which points against injury being a cause. Injury can be on both sides, but the resultant deformities would probably be different. The deformity in the top picture, dislocated knees, could be caused non-accidentally by downward force on the upper leg and upward force on the lower leg. However, the resultant tearing of ligaments and soft tissues would be extensive, causing marked swelling and exquisite tenderness of the knee joints. If such 'injuries' are painless, the child happy and the limb movable, it suggests that either the injury is old and the acute damage has resolved or that it is a natural deformity. The deformities in the lower pictures could only result from gross violence as the infant foot is highly mobile. Natural remodelling with time, would correct any deformity, unless the feet were held in the broken position, which would imply major psychiatric problems in the perpetrator.

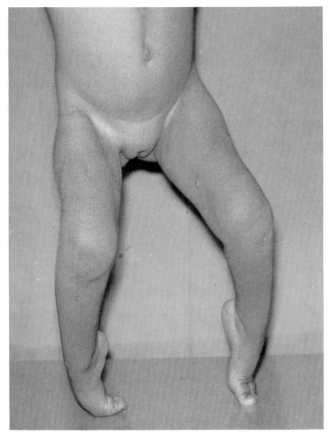

Fig. 88 Deformities caused by muscle imbalance. The position of our limbs is dependent on the tension of different muscle groups attached to each limb. Each movement requires certain muscle groups to contract and the antagonistic groups to relax. Even at rest, however, there is still tension in the muscles maintaining the position of the limb. If imbalance of power occurs between opposing muscles, for example if one set loses power, such as in polio, the opposing muscles act alone on the limb and the limb position becomes abnormal. This occurs slowly, and so limb position and the deformity will alter with time. The muscle groups may become spastic as seen in some brain-damaged children, all the muscles having increasing tension, but in the leg, for example, those muscles keeping the leg straight predominate, so the leg becomes fixed and the foot also points downwards. If sporadic groups of muscles are affected, the resultant deformities will be asymmetrical, but painless.

83

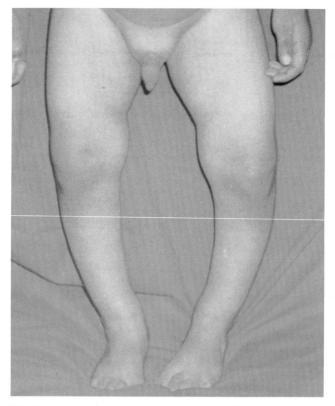

Fig. 89 Bow legs caused by rickets. Fractures of the legs followed by movement of the bone-ends cause limb deformities. A common type of accidental fracture in toddlers is the 'greenstick' fracture, when only one side of the bone is broken, the other side remaining intact, as happens when trying to snap a fresh twig. Swelling may occur, but deformity is not marked. However, non-accidental injuries are commonly a result of a direct blow to the limb, causing the bone to break straight across. This allows movement and, therefore, can produce deformity. Even in severely displaced bone-ends after fracture, remodelling is so efficient, that long-term deformities rarely occur. This child shows bowing of the legs and swelling of the ankles, symmetrically. He is also standing, which is painful even with 'greenstick' fractures. Rickets is becoming more common in Britain, often in immigrant populations, but still occurs in the indigenous population. There are several causes of rickets, but nutritional deficiency is still the commonest. The deformities may not, therefore, be the direct result of non-accidental injury, but the rickets may be caused by neglect.

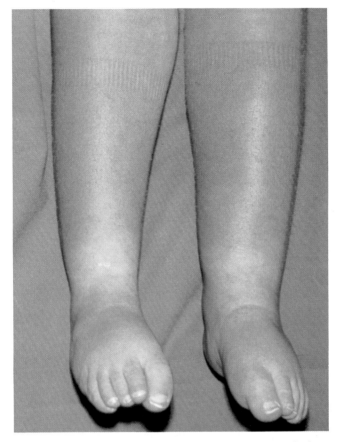

Fig. 90 Fracture of the leg. The legs of this child are asymmetrical with swelling occurring in the lower part of the left leg. The fracture allows bleeding from the bone, and damage to the tissues by sharp pieces of bone causes further swelling. The trauma causing the fracture may also have injured the muscle, again producing swelling. The area would be tender and the child would resist any attempts to move the limb. Most accidental fractures in the school age child are spiral and are frequently caused by rotational forces, such as attempting to turn on the leg whilst the foot is fixed. Non-accidental fractures are usually caused by direct blows to the limb. The considerable force required would cause bruising of the overlying skin, however, blood from the accidentally fractured bone can track along to the skin and also cause bruising. An explanation consistent with the required violence must be sought. Vague, improbable or implausible explanations should raise suspicion.

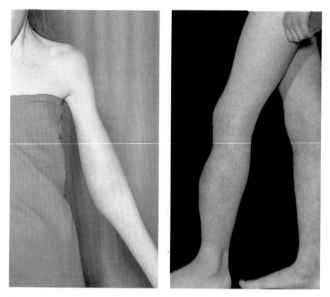

Fig. 91 Asymmetrical swellings. These figures show examples of naturally occurring asymmetrical deformities. In the left picture the swelling is caused by a bone tumour, the arm may be painful to use and the swelling tender when touched. It is quite possible that no bruising will be present. Any malignant tumour such as this is likely to cause constitutional symptoms, such as weight loss, malaise, lethargy and poor appetite. However, a child who has been subjected to both physical and psychological abuse or neglect, may also have a poor appetite, weight loss and be lethargic from depression.
The picture on the right shows a muscle disorder which causes swelling of the muscle. There is no limitation of movement, no tenderness and the child is standing. This would be impossible with the degree of damage to the leg necessary to simulate this abnormality.

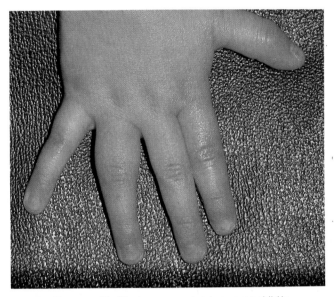

Fig. 92   Osteomyelitis. The immune system in a young child is immature, so infections can gain a foothold readily. This infant has an isolated asymmetrical swelling of a finger due to an infection of the bone (osteomyelitis). There is no inflammation of the overlying skin, which is more consistent with a fracture than osteomyelitis. This is because tuberculosis is the causative disease, and does not provoke inflammation. Although not a common childhood disease, the incidence of tuberculosis is increasing with the enlarging immigrant population. Certain races, predominantly African, suffer from a blood disorder (sickle cell disease) which can cause exactly the same swelling of the finger. Inflammation will, again, not be marked. The child with osteomyelitis or sickle cell disease may have constitutional symptoms such as a fever, but there may be little to aid distinction between naturally occurring disease and NAI.

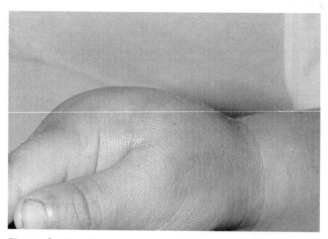

Fig. 93 Swelling of the back of the hand. The infant is unlikely to possess sufficient power to cause an injury producing this degree of swelling. If the child is not suffering from a generalised disease, then this injury would have been caused by outside agents. If the child is mobile, slammed doors or dropped heavy objects are possible explanations, if the child is not mobile, this degree of injury becomes more sinister. Any explanation must include violence, accidental or otherwise. Small fragments of bone torn from the ends of the long bones by excessive longitudinal force, such as suddenly jerking the child up by his hands, will show no external markers such as this. Nevertheless such fractures are painful and the child may scream if the limb is touched. Other causes of this behaviour, especially if the infant is old enough to recognise and dislike strangers, should be sought before a fracture is considered.

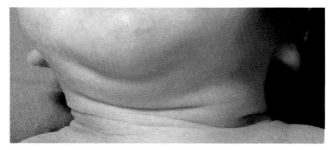

Fig. 94 Lump in the neck. The neck is a relatively well protected part of the toddler's anatomy and even in non-accidental beating, the neck is frequently spared. Injuries in this area are, consequently, less likely to have occurred accidentally. This lump was caused by the muscle being torn during delivery, and several months may elapse before the swelling is resorbed. Tearing of the muscle requires considerable force, and if not caused by birth injury, a suitable explanation must be sought. Neck swellings such as a goitre, are quite common, so it is useful to attempt to determine the origin of the lump. A lump in the thyroid gland, for example, would be naturally occurring. One in a muscle may have been caused by trauma.

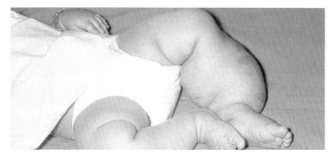

Fig. 95 Asymmetrical swelling of the leg. If presented with a child who appears to have suffered a terrible injury, it is good practice to hazard a guess at the cause, considering the site of the injury and age of the child. The explanation must then be consistent with the deformity. This infant shows a huge swelling of the leg and bruising over the area. Such a deformity is not likely to be the result of massive bleeding caused by violence. Such bleeding would virtually exsanguinate the child who would appear pale and life-less. The deformity would also be exquisitely tender. If the child is happy and alert whilst sporting such a mass, then major trauma is excluded. It is not sufficient for a parental explanation to be dismissed as implausible and action taken, the investigator must offer an alternative, more plausible explanation himself if he wishes to disprove the story of the accused.

Poisoning

Only a few cases of deliberate poisoning of children have been reported and the problem has only been recognised for the past few years.

Many agents have been used including drugs that either parent possessed or common household items such as salt. This form of NAI is very worrying and several cases have ended in death. The aggressor is often extremely adept at concealing the true origin of the child's illness and often the diagnosis is reached only after the child has been subjected to repeated hospital admissions, and multiple investigations. Many theories have been advanced as to the cause of this problem including marital conflicts, projection of anxieties and unresolved grief. However, whatever the cause, once the diagnosis is established, careful psychiatric care is indicated.

Early recognition of this problem is extremely difficult. Many children accidentally poison themselves; those children too young to have acquired the poison themselves may have been fed by an obliging sibling! However, certain aspects should alert the observer: repeated poisonings over a period, possibly with admissions to different hospitals, repeated hospital admissions with bizarre symptoms and no diagnosis, and the unexplained death of another sibling with symptoms similar to the child in question. It must be remembered that repeated bizarre behaviour may be the result of epilepsy or other organic disorders and an unexplained death with the same symptoms may be the result of a genetically inherited disease.

A related form of 'battering' is falsifying an illness. The child may be admitted repeatedly for investigations of an illness, only to find that all symptoms disappear when the mother is excluded from the bedside. Instances of this problem include falsifying recurrent temperatures by placing the thermometer in a cup of tea or hot water bottle or contaminating samples such as urine, with blood or bacteria. Parents may be adept at avoiding detection and the observer must be alert to repeated inconclusive hospital admissions. The following are case histories of some such children:

A four year old girl was admitted unconscious and fitting. The fits were controlled and over the next few days the child made a complete recovery, all investigations having shown her to be normal. Both parents denied possessing any drugs other than aspirin, which were kept in a locked cabinet. The child was then readmitted twice over the next eight weeks with drowsiness, poor co-ordination and a staggering gait. She recovered rapidly with no sequelae and again results of all investigations were normal. Six weeks after the last discharge she was admitted deeply unconscious and died from a heart attack. High concentrations of an antidepressant were found in the stomach and blood. Mother had been depressed since the birth of another baby, and had been on this antidepressant for the last nine months.

A six week old child was admitted in a state of dehydration. Investigation revealed a high blood salt. The child was treated and made a rapid recovery. Over the next few months the child was repeatedly admitted with dehydration or drowsiness, and each time the blood salt was high. Eventually mother admitted giving the child excess salt and had psychiatric treatment. Nevertheless, at the age of 14 months, the child was admitted in coma and died; the blood salt was found to be extremely high.

A six year old girl was admitted for investigation of foul smelling, bloody urine. At the age of eight months she had been diagnosed as having a urinary tract infection and had been on continuous antibiotics ever since. She had had multiple admissions for investigation which included X-rays, and exploratory operations, all of which were inconclusive. Eventually it was discovered that the mother suffered from a chronic urinary tract infection, and had been adding her own urine to that of the child. The child was then found to be entirely normal, but not until she had been subjected to many unpleasant experiences.

These three cases illustrate some aspects of the problem of non-accidental poisoning and 'battering by proxy'. In some cases it is impossible for the outside observer to differentiate abuse from genuine illness, but a knowledge of the social and psychological stresses within the family, and evidence of repeated admissions to hospital may raise doubts.

Deprivation

Deprivation may be either physical or psychological (the so-called 'soft battering'), although frequently elements of both exist concurrently. All the children in the family may be deprived, but, curiously, often only one is singled out and excluded from the family circle. This child may be the result of an unwanted pregnancy, may have been premature and so separated from the mother at birth, or separation may have been inevitable from repeated hospital admissions. Commonly, however, there is no obvious reason for the maltreatment of this particular child. The child may be physically excluded from the rest of the family, being shut in a separate room, siblings may be forbidden to talk or play with him, and only the bare minimum of food allowed. This situation continues with the concurrence of the rest of the family, indeed, the sufferer may believe his lot in life to be normal.

Psychological deprivation within an ostensibly normal family is most difficult to detect and may manifest itself only after years of deprivation, when the child may be severely disturbed. Emotional deprivation per se may not be intended. If the family is ambitious, only repeated success may be rewarded, so the child who does not achieve as highly as expected, may be subjected to continual disapproval, whilst actually requiring love and encouragement. Conversely, the child may just be ignored. The toddler may fail to thrive, despite being fed adequately, or be excessively friendly to adults whilst showing no signs of pleasure on recognising his parents. In hospital, this may be seen when a child enjoys his new environment and demands attention from everybody, whereas a normal child will be distraught at his mother's apparent desertion. The school-age child may fail at school or become disobedient or aggressive in an attempt to gain some form of attention, however unpleasant the consequences. The adolescent may run away from home, be excessively demanding, or extreme cases may attempt suicide. However, not all children exhibiting such behaviour do so from deprivation.

Physical deprivation may be more easily detected. The infant may be malnourished (Fig. 96) from inadequate intake of food. The child may be small for his age and apathetic, However, chronic intestinal or chest disease

(Fig. 97), may render a child virtually cadaveric despite a normal or increased appetite.

The child may be left for days in the same nappy and clothes with no attention paid to hygiene or general cleanliness. This may cause repeated episodes of gastroenteritis or other infections.

A child is easily scrubbed clean before the health visitor calls, or for the trip to the baby clinic, but if the nappy has been left on constantly, a severe erosive nappy rash will develop (Fig. 98), which is difficult to disguise. However, nappy rashes are also commonly seen in well cared for infants, and certain skin diseases such as eczema or seborrhoeic dermatitis predispose the infant to a severe nappy rash (Fig. 99), which may be resistant to careful treatment. If there is concern about the child, further evidence of neglect or battering should be sought. The child in Fig. 98 had been left clothed only in a nappy in an unheated room and developed frostbite and gangrene of the hand (Fig. 100).

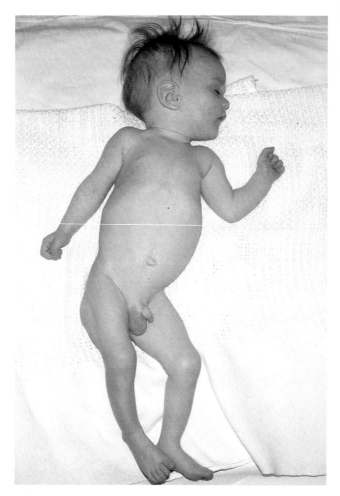

Fig. 96 Deprivation syndrome. A small child is totally dependent on outside agents for all his requirements, including food. Thus, a child who receives inappropriate or inadequate food will fail to thrive. The child's length and weight will be considerably below that expected for his age, however, the head circumference may well be normal as brain growth is preserved at the expense of other organs. The child will be apathetic, limp, have no facial expression and will respond to discomfort with only a whimper. The limbs are thin and may be cold from poor circulation through the skin, the buttocks are wasted and the hair is fine and sparse. Rapid weight gain following feeding usually excludes serious underlying disease.

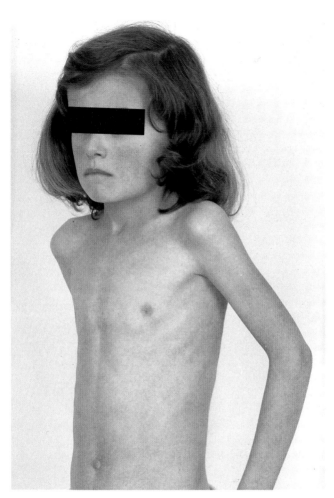

Fig. 97 Chronic disease. Chronic disease may cause growth problems in childhood and the child may be painfully thin. A common intestinal disease (coeliac disease) occurs when wheat-containing food is introduced into the diet. The infant may lose weight rapidly and become intensely miserable, resembling a deprived child. Inadequate absorption of food often produces a prominent abdomen, which is not seen in the starved child. Chronic disease affecting any body system, such as the chest, shown here, or the kidneys, may cause extreme wasting. The child, however, is less likely to be apathetic, he will be pleased to see his family and react with them and, even if offered an adequate diet, will fail to gain weight.

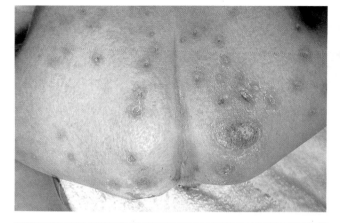

Fig. 98 Neglect. The grimy evidence of neglect of personal hygiene can largely be scrubbed away, if visitors are expected. Bacteria in the faeces react with urine to produce ammonia, which is highly irritant. Initially the nappy area becomes red and inflamed, however, the skin creases between the thighs and the genital area are usually spared. If the nappy area is not carefully tended at this stage, blistering occurs and then ulceration, as seen here. This is more difficult to hide and to explain satisfactorily. The ulcers shown in both these illustrations are multiple, large and deep, which implies that the process has been going on for some time. Not all severe nappy rash is neglect (vide infra). The mother herself may not worry about her own personal hygiene and therefore, not be too concerned about her infant, or the mother may be inexperienced and be unable to cope with the demands made by the arrival of a helpless infant. Again, the entire social circumstance should be considered.

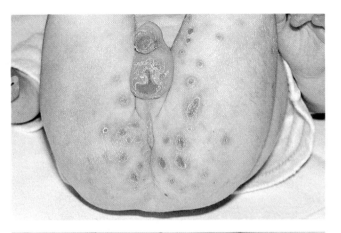

Fig. 99 Skin disease. These brothers both have infantile eczema. Skin disease can predispose the child to severe nappy rash. If the skin is itchy, the child will scratch, break the skin barrier and allow infection. The disease itself may cause fissuring and cracking of the skin, again facilitating bacterial invasion and a severe ulcerated nappy rash. A skin disease will frequently affect other areas of the body, which will aid differentiation. The chronically sick child commonly has a reduced immunity, so infection in the nappy area may then spread more rapidly than in the normal child. The nappy rash in these figures is not as extensive as in Fig. 98, the ulcers are smaller and shallower, and several are healing, which suggests attempts at care are being made. These differences can not be relied on, however, to help differentiation.

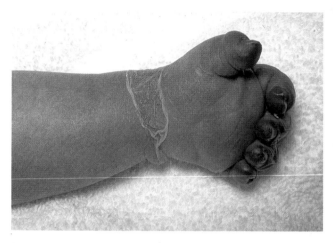

Fig. 100 Frostbite and gangrene. This is an extreme example of deprivation. The child was left, clothed only in a nappy in an unheated room. The limbs are more affected than the trunk as, to conserve heat, the circulation to the extremities is diverted to deeper structures and to vital organs, such as the brain, heart and kidneys. This child must have been left in the cold for some hours. This demonstrates, however, the importance of examining the child carefully for any other markers of non-accidental injury or neglect. Superficial skin infection, especially around the nose, excoriation of the upper lip from persistent nasal discharge, diarrhoea or chronic cough may be signs of neglect. They also happen as frequently in loving and caring families.

Index
Entries in **bold** refer to Fig. numbers